T0298460

Human Relations and Hospital Care

Originally published in 1964, this book describes the hospital service as it is seen by patients. It is based mainly on interviews with a random sample of patients and discusses the relationships between patients and between them and hospital doctors, nurses, and general practitioners. The best available medical care should not only be given, but the patient and his relatives should feel that this has been given. Explanations need to be seen not as a lavish appendage, but as an integral part of medical care. Recognition and acceptance of this responsibility could stimulate interest in patients' social lives, so that hospital staff become more aware of the difficulties patients may encounter when they leave hospital. This in turn could lead to greater integration between the hospital and welfare services and between the hospital and the general practitioners. Still relevant today this study can now be read in its historical context.

Human Relations and Hospital Care

Ann Cartwright

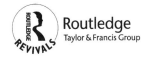

Routledge
Taylor & Francis Group

First published in 1964
by Routledge & Kegan Paul

This edition first published in 2024 by Routledge
4 Park Square, Milton Park, Abingdon, Oxon, OX14 4RN

and by Routledge
605 Third Avenue, New York, NY 10017

Routledge is an imprint of the Taylor & Francis Group, an informa business

© 1964 Institute of Community Studies (a division of The Young Foundation)

Publisher's Note
The publisher has gone to great lengths to ensure the quality of this reprint but points out that some imperfections in the original copies may be apparent.

Disclaimer
The publisher has made every effort to trace copyright holders and welcomes correspondence from those they have been unable to contact.

A Library of Congress record exists under LCCN: 65007583

ISBN: 978-1-032-54312-3 (hbk)
ISBN: 978-1-003-42515-1 (ebk)
ISBN: 978-1-032-54492-2 (pbk)

Book DOI 10.4324/9781003425151

HUMAN RELATIONS
AND
HOSPITAL CARE

★

Ann Cartwright

LONDON
ROUTLEDGE & KEGAN PAUL

First published 1964
by Routledge & Kegan Paul Limited
Broadway House, 68–74 Carter Lane
London, E.C.4

Reprinted 1969

Printed in Great Britain by
Lowe & Brydone (Printers) Ltd., London

SBN 7100 3919 0

CONTENTS

v

Contents

TABLES

Tables

viii

Tables

ix

ACKNOWLEDGEMENTS

M Y colleagues and I are grateful for the support received from the Nuffield Provincial Hospitals Trust for the main study and to the Joseph Rowntree Memorial Trust for a grant which covered the cost of the preliminary inquiries. We collaborated from the start with a committee under the chairmanship of Professor Norman Morris, which had been set up with the co-operation of the National Association for Mental Health to promote such a study as this, and we had the advice and encouragement of the committee throughout the research. Rosalind Marshall and Wyn Tucker helped at all stages—with the sampling, coding, analysis, and preparation of the final report. Maurice Backett, Margot Jefferys, Peter Marris, Michael Warren, Peter Willmott, and Michael Young read the various questionnaires and drafts, suggesting many improvements. The patients were interviewed by Angela Adams, Jean Brent, Muriel Donald, Josephine Goodey, Elizabeth Grabham, Patricia Haward, Rosalind Marshall, and Chris West. Others who helped in various ways were Brian Abel-Smith, Derek Allcorn, John Brotherston, Gwen Cartwright, Edmund Cooney, J. O. F. Davies, Gordon Forsyth, Sheila Gray, John Horder, Dilys Kahn, Ronald Mac Keith, Nicolas Malleson, Fred Martin, Winifred Raphael, R. W. Revans, Margaret Scott Wright, Marjorie Simpson, Mervyn Susser, L. R. S. Titley, Richard Titmuss, Phyllis Willmott, other colleagues at the Institute of Community Studies, and the members of the Institute's Advisory Committee. I am indebted to all these, and to the patients, the general practitioners and the secretaries of the Hospital Management Committees, who made this study possible.

PART ONE

Introductory

I

BACKGROUND
TO THE STUDY

THE successful application of medical knowledge depends on what patients think and feel about doctors, nurses, and hospitals. A patient's decision to become one, his willingness to be examined, his acceptance of treatment, depend on his confidence in the skill and humanity of doctors and nurses and on his feelings about the institution where he may be treated.

This book describes the hospital service as it is seen by patients. It is based mainly on interviews with a random[1] sample of patients and discusses the relationships between patients and between them and hospital doctors, nurses, and general practitioners. The views of a small sample of general practitioners have also been obtained.

There are a number of obvious limitations in an interview survey like this. What people say is never more (and may be less) than a part of the truth. Patients may report facts inaccurately either because they wish to mislead or because they do not recall the facts clearly themselves. There are techniques for reducing certain errors and some of the findings of a survey like this can be checked by comparison with information collected in other ways. But the danger remains. There are even more pitfalls about opinions, as distinct from facts. It is, for instance, very difficult to measure the strength of an opinion, and yet this may be crucial. Some opinions given in response to specific questions may be so lightly held that they are better regarded as random whims. Another problem is that opinions may be, obviously often are, based on misinterpretation of fact. It should be said that, with this survey, even where this was suspected, the opinions have been reported all the same—for they can well illustrate the

[1] Random is used here in the statistical sense. It implies not that patients were chosen haphazardly, but that each one had an equal chance of being included in the sample.

kinds of misunderstanding which arise, or suggest ways in which these might be avoided.

A further danger is that people may give the answer they feel the interviewer wants them to give. There may also be a tendency to reduce complexity to black or white—a kind of distortion to which this sort of study is probably particularly prone. Patients who have been treated in hospital, and have returned home cured or helped, are likely to feel grateful. The hospital may acquire a halo. Alternatively, a strong feeling of dissatisfaction about one feature of their care may bias them against everything. Another limitation of this approach is that patients are not able to assess the clinical efficiency of their hospital treatment. They may think it successful or unsuccessful, but they cannot know whether other forms of treatment would have been more appropriate, involving fewer risks or less discomfort.

But patients' comments on the way they are treated as people are relevant to any general evaluation of the hospital service. They are important not simply as an index of consumer satisfaction—indeed, it can be held that 'consumer protection geared to consumer satisfaction could lead to the sacrifice of good medical treatment for the sake of avoiding complaints'[1]—but because effective medical care depends on patients' attitudes and co-operation.

Methods

Every year three million men and women in England and Wales leave their homes and families to go into hospital. The initial problem was to obtain a sample of these people. It was decided to interview them in their own homes rather than in hospital, because they were more likely to talk freely there and could also discuss their experiences after they had left hospital. Although some hospitals might have been prepared to give us the necessary information about a sample of their patients, others might not, and this would have introduced an important bias. At the same time, to approach the patients through selected hospitals might have led people to identify the interviewers with the hospitals and to fear that their comments might be conveyed back to the hospital staff.

The method used to obtain a sample of patients largely overcomes these difficulties. The study was carried out in 12 randomly selected districts in England and Wales. Every twenty-second person on the electoral register in each of these was written to and asked whether he or she had been in hospital in the last six months. Eighty-seven per cent of the 29,400 people who were approached in this way replied. Those who said they had been in hospital during the study period

¹ *Lancet:* 'Annotation'. Full details about all references are in Appendix 7.

4

were visited in their homes.[1] Eighty-one per cent of those who were eligible, 739 patients, were interviewed. Further details of the way the sample was selected and of the response are given in Appendix 1. A comparison between data from this inquiry and the study of hospital in-patients carried out by the Ministry of Health and General Register Office shows that the estimated hospitalization rate from this inquiry is about 11% too low. For the age and sex of patients, diagnosis, length of stay and type of hospital, the sample is reasonably representative.

A structured questionnaire was used for the interviews. A copy is in Appendix 3. Much of the information sought was for statistical analysis, but people were also asked to give examples and to elaborate their replies. This material has been used for illustration.

In addition to the patients, a sample of 144 general practitioners, 12 in each of the study areas, was selected from lists of doctors practising in the districts. Of these doctors, 124 or 86%, were interviewed. They gave their views on the relationships between hospitals and general practitioners in the particular areas, and discussed problems of communication between hospitals and general practitioners and between hospitals and patients. A copy of this interview schedule is also in Appendix 3, and more details of the sample are in Appendix 2.

The districts

The areas chosen for this study were 12 of the 547 parliamentary constituencies in England and Wales. The salient characteristics of the districts are described here and to do this they are considered in five groups.

The various factors taken into account in forming the groups are shown in Appendix 4.

1. *Middle-class town-and-country districts.* Three of the 12 constituencies—Melton in Leicestershire, Lewes in East Sussex and St. Albans in Hertfordshire—are alike in being partly rural and relatively middle class, and in having expanding populations. All three areas have a high proportion of jurors on the electoral register, a characteristic associated with property with a high rateable value.[2] All returned a Conservative Member to Parliament in 1959, and both Lewes and Melton might be described as solidly Conservative, with majorities of over 12,000. St. Albans has a rather lower majority, 8,500, and returned a Labour member in 1945. St. Albans is within commuting distance of London, a number of people in Lewes travel to and from Brighton to work and a few to London, and parts of

---

[1] A few people, 15, or 2%, were still in hospital and were seen there.
[2] Gray, P. G., Corlett, T., and Jones, P., *The Proportion of Jurors as an Index of the Economic Status of a District.*

5

Melton constituency lie within easy reach of Leicester. The populations in all three areas expanded by about a fifth between 1951 and 1961, and between 1931 and 1951 the populations in Lewes and Melton expanded by a quarter and that of St. Albans by over a half. *St. Albans* constituency consists of St. Albans Municipal Borough, an industrial, commercial, and ecclesiastical centre, and a large part of the surrounding rural district including Wheathampstead, Sandridge, and London Colney. Industries, which are varied, include aircraft, printing, electronics, electrical and general engineering, and the manufacture of nylon stockings, edible fats, musical instruments, cardboard boxes, and stained glass. *Lewes* constituency extends from Lewes Municipal Borough southwards to the sea at Newhaven Urban District and Seaford Urban District, north-west to Burgess Hill, and includes the villages of Cuckfield, Hurstpierpoint, Keymer, and Fulking. A relatively high proportion of people aged 65 and over live in this constituency, 15·3% in 1951 compared with 11% in the country as a whole. *Melton* covers Melton Mowbray Urban District and the three rural districts of Barrow-upon-Soar, Billesdon, and Melton and Belvoir. It is a large area of about 350 square miles, and extends towards the boundaries of Leicester, Loughborough, and Grantham. Though a number of people in the area work in Leicester, there are a few industries in Melton Mowbray itself, including animal feeding stuffs and engineering research laboratories, and the traditional manufacture of pork pies and Stilton cheeses. Most of the constituency is gently undulating country, on which people farm and hunt.

2. *Middle-class urban areas.* Wallasey County Borough in Cheshire and Wimbledon Municipal Borough in Surrey, the two areas in this category, have relatively static populations. Both have a high proportion of jurors and are solidly Conservative. Wimbledon is part of the Greater London area, while Wallasey is in part a dormitory suburb of Liverpool and Birkenhead. Although *Wallasey County Borough* is a single administrative area, it is made up of a number of different centres: New Brighton, Egremont, Seacombe, Liscard, and Wallasey village. It is at the tip of the Wirral, and New Brighton and Seacombe are on the River Mersey, with ferries to Liverpool. Wallasey is not so well-to-do as Wimbledon—the proportion of professional people living there in 1951 was 4·5% in the former area compared with 8·9% in the latter—while the proportion of semi-skilled and unskilled people in Wimbledon was lower than in any of the other areas in our inquiry. *Wimbledon* is largely a residential borough and has little industry. The few firms are small and mostly occupied with light engineering and metalwork. There are many green areas besides the Common and Wimbledon Park, and these open spaces together cover about a third of the total area.

Background to the Study

3. *Agricultural area*. *Torrington* in Devon is the only agricultural constituency in the study. It is a large area of nearly 600 square miles going from Bideford Municipal Borough and Northam Urban District on the north coast to Crediton Urban District and Okehampton Municipal Borough on the fringes of Dartmoor, and covering several rural districts. There are many agricultural workers in this area, the proportion of jurors is fairly low, and, although the constituency returned a Conservative M.P. in 1959, his majority was not high. Previously there had been a Liberal member. The population in the rural part of the area declined by about 4% between 1951 and 1961, but this was largely offset by increases in the urban districts, particularly Crediton.

4. *Working-class towns*. The three constituencies here—Leigh in Lancashire, Pontypool in Monmouthshire, and Durham—are all small, relatively homogeneous towns. *Leigh* comprises Leigh Municipal Borough, Atherton Urban District, and Tyldesley Urban District. Mining, cotton, and more recently light engineering are the main industries. *Pontypool* constituency covers the top part of the most eastern of the Welsh mining valleys and consists of Blaenavon Urban District, at the head of the valley, Pontypool Urban District, and Cwmbran Urban District. The chief industries are mining, iron and steel works, and nylon spinning. *Durham* constituency covers Durham Municipal Borough, Spennymoor Urban District, Hetton Urban District, and Durham Rural District. Both Hetton-le-Hole and Spennymoor are mining towns whose populations are now declining. Durham Rural District contains one or two large mining villages such as Coxhoe.

Two of these districts, Durham Municipal Borough and Cwmbran Urban District, are very different from the others. Durham has a University College, a castle and a cathedral with attractive precincts, but this is only a small area, and Durham Municipal Borough as a whole contains less than a quarter of the constituency's population. The distinctive feature of Cwmbran is that a New Town is being developed there. Between 1951 and 1961 its population expanded by nearly two-thirds, whereas that of Blaenavon, which is at the head of the same valley, declined by 14%. All three constituencies have a very low proportion of jurors on the electoral register, under 2%, and are solidly Labour.

5. *Working-class city districts*. Sunderland North, Lambeth Vauxhall, and Birmingham Sparkbrook are the three constituencies in this group. Birmingham Sparkbrook is a marginal seat, and the Labour majority in Sunderland North is under 2,500. So of the three, only Lambeth Vauxhall can be described as solidly Labour, though even here the majority is under 8,000. Since all three are only part of

administrative districts, statistics are not available for the constituencies themselves, but only for the areas of which these constituencies are part. These areas contain a fairly low proportion of people in professional or intermediate occupations, but not so low as in Leigh, Durham, and Pontypool.

Sunderland North covers all the parts of Sunderland on the north side of the River Wear and a number of wards on the south side which border on the river. This area includes the shipbuilding yards and also the seaside resort of Roker. *Birmingham Sparkbrook* is a wedge-shaped area lying mostly between the main Warwick and Stratford roads. In the narrow half of the wedge nearer the centre of Birmingham live three broad groups of people; those who have come to Birmingham recently, including people from Ireland and the West Indies, older residents who moved in as young married couples and are now in their fifties and sixties, and retail traders. Further out, in Foxhollies, there are more semi-detached houses and a generally suburban atmosphere. There are a number of big factories in the area, Joseph Lucas, Rover, B.S.A., and Singer, and several smaller ones making such varied things as bedding, buttons, air conditioning, gas equipment, and kirby grips. *Lambeth Vauxhall* consists of six wards of Lambeth Metropolitan Borough, and lies between Waterloo Bridge and Vauxhall Bridge on the south side of the River Thames. It was heavily bombed during the 1939–45 war. A rebuilding programme has been under way during the last few years; old and derelict houses, wharves and warehouses have been replaced by modern blocks of flats and office buildings.

Thus the districts studied included parts of cities, a new town, villages, seaside resorts, suburbs, a mining valley, and a cathedral precinct. What of the patients who lived in these places?

The patients, their illnesses, and the hospitals

Just under two-thirds of the patients were women. Nearly half, 45%, were under 45 and about a fifth were aged 65 or more. (Their age and sex distribution is shown in detail in Appendix 1, Table H.) The majority, 78%, were married, 10% were single, and 12% widowed or divorced. Two-thirds of the men were working full time before they went into hospital. Less than a fifth of the women did so, and a tenth worked part time.

Sixteen per cent of the patients had gone into hospital for the delivery of a baby, 47% were surgical patients,[1] and the remaining 37% medical ones. Patients' descriptions of their conditions have

[1] Surgical patients means simply those who had an operation, who are not necessarily the same as those treated in surgical wards.

8

been classified according to the International Statistical Classification of Diseases, Injuries and Causes of Death.[1] The proportions with different diseases and symptoms are given in Appendix 1, Table I, which also shows the distribution based on hospital records from the Ministry of Health and General Register Office inquiry. The proportion of patients with many conditions was similar on the two inquiries, but comparatively few malignant diseases were recorded on this study. Some of these patients may have died before they could be interviewed and others may have been too ill to participate. In addition, some patients may not know when they have had cancer, while others may be reluctant to talk about it. One interviewer described an example of the latter:

> When I asked Mrs. A, 'What were you in hospital for?' there was a slight pause before she said she had had a radical mastectomy. She then sat watching me, as though looking for my reaction. It was evident that she hated telling me this, and the thought of it still worried her deeply. It was impossible to ask the next question, 'What was the name of your condition?' When there was no reaction from me and I did not ask for further details she became less reserved, and later glad to discuss her sense of shock when she discovered she had had a radical. 'The G.P. thought it was mastitis—a common complaint in a woman of my age. I was quite convinced I was going in for a minor job. It was a great shock to me. The houseman didn't come for two days. The sister didn't tell me either. I did feel somebody could have spared just two minutes to explain! I can see now that it had to be but I wasn't very happy about it at the time.'

It was obvious that part of the shock was lying fearing that radical mastectomy indicated a malignant growth, and facing that fact alone. 'Personally I would much rather be told about things than lie and worry. To me the known is much better than the unknown. I would have liked things explained more—although they knew that I and my husband were in touch with my own doctor, who really explained things very fully. I did ask the sister once or twice—little things—and she'd say: 'Ask Mr. B. when he comes in." Well, these surgeons haven't the time and you can't discuss things as fully as you'd like. They're at the foot of the bed and on to the next patient before you know.

'Mr. B. said, "Don't worry. We'll find out when we get the results from the path. lab." But it was my own doctor who explained that six weeks later.'

There was a pause each time she mentioned the path. report. Talking about it at all was painful for her. It was not until nearly the end of the interview that she told me she had had post-operative deep X-ray as an out-patient at —— hospital (a cancer hospital). She again watched my reaction when she mentioned this hospital. It was quite impossible for

[1] World Health Organization, *Manual of the International Statistical Classification of Diseases, Injuries and Causes of Death.*

her to say 'They found it was malignant—I had cancer.' She knew that I realized the nature of her condition.

Rather less than half of the patients were in hospital for between one and three weeks. Nearly a quarter were in for less than a week, and a fifth for a month or more.

The patients had been in 199 different hospitals[1]. Three-quarters of the patients were in general acute ones, 9% in maternity, women's or gynaecological, 3% chronic or long-stay, 3% T.B., chest or isolation, 3% mental illness, and the remaining 8% in miscellaneous hospitals.

Eleven per cent were in hospitals with under 50 beds and at the other extreme 17% in ones with 500 or more. Eleven per cent of the patients were in teaching hospitals and 3% had gone in as private, fee-paying patients. One only had an amenity bed.

Plan of the book

The efficiency of hospitals depends on what happens outside them as well as inside. If people do not arrive there until their illness is too far advanced, the hospital is not functioning as effectively as it might. So this book starts in Part I by looking at the delays and difficulties patients had before they were admitted. It then describes, in Part II, the day-to-day life in the hospital ward.

Communications between patients and hospital staff are discussed in Part III, which explores patients' desire for explanations, their sources of information and some ways in which communications might be improved. Then there is an account in Part IV of the problems encountered by the patients when they left hospital and returned to their families, homes and jobs. Finally Part V discusses some of the ways in which patients' attitudes and experiences vary, according to the sort of hospital they go into, the reason for which they are admitted, and their own background.

The majority of patients were satisfied with the medical treatment they received in hospital and had nothing but praise for the nurses and the way they looked after them. In view of this it may seem that too much attention has been paid to the patients who were dissatisfied. Statistical analysis should put these criticisms in perspective, and when particular emphasis is put on the shortcomings of the service, this is in the hope that more can be learnt from the occasional criticisms than from the general chorus of praise.

[1] The hospitals attended by the patients in our sample can be regarded as a cluster sample of hospitals. The chance of any hospital being included is proportional to the number of discharges, since those attended by one patient in the sample are included once, those by two twice, etc. Data about the hospitals were obtained from the *Hospital Year Book 1961*.

But there is one inevitable bias in this study about which nothing can be done. The views of the patients who died in hospital, or soon after they came out, are not included. The numbers are not inconsiderable; about 200,000 people die in our hospitals each year, and deaths account for about 7% of all adult 'discharges'. This study is confined to the 93% who came out of hospital alive.

II

ADMISSION TO HOSPITAL

THE value of the hospital service depends not only on the quality of medical care, but also on how patients are selected. This survey shows the routes by which patients got into hospital, and illustrates the various delays and barriers that can come between the patient and the hospital bed. But, of course, we only interviewed patients who were admitted to hospital, and it may not always be those who are most in need of this care who receive it. For example, preliminary analyses of the recent Perinatal Mortality Survey[1] showed that less than half the mothers with severe toxaemia were admitted to hospital for the necessary treatment, and 70% of patients having their fifth or subsequent babies (carrying a 60% increased risk to the baby) were booked for confinement outside hospital. Our interviews with general practitioners suggest that this problem is not entirely confined to maternity patients.

The chapter starts with a brief description of how patients go into hospital. Some are taken ill suddenly and go in straight away. For others the process is more complex, involving several stages and different people. The various possible sources of delay are discussed in turn, starting with the patient himself, then the general practitioner, and after that the hospital. Next the chapter discusses the views of general practitioners on hospital delays, views which are, in some ways, more illuminating than those of patients and which emphasize the importance of the relationship between general practitioners and hospital staff. Finally, some ways of reducing delays are considered.

How patients were admitted

The part played by general practitioners in referring patients to hospital is shown in Table 1. The great majority of patients, 88%, were sent to hospital by their own doctor. For 28% the general practitioner arranged for the patient to be admitted directly to hospital,

[1] National Birthday Trust Fund.

56% were seen first at the out-patient department, and the remaining 4% were visited in their homes by a consultant under the National Health Service domiciliary consultation arrangements.[1]

TABLE 1

THE GENERAL PRACTITIONER AND ADMISSION TO HOSPITAL

	%
Referred by general practitioner	
Admitted directly	28⎫
Seen at out-patients	56 ⎬88
Domiciliary consultation	4⎭
General practitioner consulted but did not refer ..	2
General practitioner not consulted	10
Number of patients (= 100%)	722

The number of people in this table is less than the 739 in the sample because information on this point was incomplete for 17 people. In some later tables, also, small numbers of people are excluded for the same reason.

Ten per cent of the patients went into hospital without consulting their general practitioner about the illness for which they were admitted. Half of these had had accidents and several of the others were taken ill suddenly. For example, one man had a coronary thrombosis and was taken to hospital from the office where he had the attack.

A number had been mentally ill. A single man of about 50 had a nervous breakdown and his brother took him straight to the hospital without going to his own doctor. A married woman suddenly forgot everything on her way to work one morning. She went up to a policeman, who took her to the infirmary, where she was admitted.

Others had been attending hospital for one condition and had had another diagnosed there. A few patients were referred to hospital by their dentist, and two maternity patients said they had gone straight to the hospital or clinic doctor without seeing their general practitioner.

A small group of patients, 2%, had consulted their general practitioner about their illness, but had not been sent to hospital by him. Most of them were admitted as emergencies when their illness became acute.

[1] Most consultants receive a fee of four guineas for these consultations, but full-time consultants receive no payment for the first eight in any quarter. There is a maximum payment of 200 guineas in any quarter.

13

Delays caused by the patient

When they were asked whether they thought they had been to their doctor as soon as it was necessary,[1] one in five of the patients said they felt they had not done so. Many of the reasons they gave for not going earlier were vague and could not be classified, but 39% of these patients said they had not realized their condition was serious, 12% gave fear or embarrassment as the reason for not going earlier, 9% family or business ties, 4% thought their doctor was too busy or otherwise unapproachable, and 2% did not think he would be able to do anything to help them.

Some of the comments from the 39% who said they did not realize what was the matter with them are given below.

'You keep putting these things off—thinking it's something you've had to eat. You take a tablet and it goes off. It always seems to come in the night and you feel you can't call the doctor in then.' (Gall bladder removed.)

'I kept thinking it would right itself. You doctor yourself and don't know what's wrong.' (Prolapse repair.)

'I didn't go to see the doctor for myself. I took my son to him. I didn't know there was anything wrong with me. I didn't even feel bad. I'd had it for six months and had been gradually losing weight. I didn't take any notice of it. He sent me straight away to the out-patients.' (Thyroidectomy.)

Others had made diagnoses which frightened them and they put off going because of this. One or two had been deterred by the thought of an operation.

'I thought it was my heart, so I was a bit scared, to tell you the truth.' (Disease of thyroid.)

'I lost my voice about October and I didn't go to the doctor because I was afraid I'd got cancer and I'd have to have an operation.' (Nervous breakdown.)

A few were embarrassed.

'I was a bit shy—but there's nothing to be shy about.' (Piles.)

'To tell you the truth I don't like anything to do with that.' (Hysterectomy.)

Nine per cent had postponed consultation for family or business reasons. 'I was studying the family. The children were taking their exams, so I put off going. Then there were comments like: 'We're not a family for bothering the doctor', 'I don't like making a fuss'.

[1] Question 5: 'Do you think you went to the doctor as soon as it was necessary?' IF NO, 'Why didn't you go earlier?' Questions about opinions are given in a footnote unless the exact form of the question is stated or implied in the text.

How much do these delays matter? Sometimes they may have had a serious effect on the development of illnesses—nine of these patients had some form of neoplasm, including one with a rodent ulcer on her face, and two who were admitted for mastectomy; ten others had a hysterectomy or a dilatation and curretage. For other patients delay may have caused discomfort and possibly some temporary disability. Eleven had had hernia operations, ten prolapse repairs, seven were suffering from varicose veins or piles and seven from ear, nose, throat or teeth conditions.

How can such delays be avoided? One way is to help people to appreciate the significance of symptoms and the range of normal variations, and to become more aware of the possibilities and limitations of modern medical care.

'I should have gone to the doctor before really, but I have piles and I thought the blood might come from there. Then I heard on the radio—the doctor in the morning—that this blood might be cancer, and a lady came on afterwards and said they could cure it, so then I went to my doctor.' (Dilatation and curettage.)

Another way to reduce these delays would be to change the relationship between some patients and their general practitioners so that they did not postpone going to see him, as they now do, because of embarrassment or dislike of bothering him. A third possibility would be for general practitioners to play a more active part in identifying undiagnosed conditions, by carrying out certain regular examinations of some patients. Backett[1] has suggested that the family doctor should be increasingly concerned with prevention and early diagnosis, and one of the possibilities he discusses is the routine examination of groups of susceptible women for pre-symptomatic cancer of the uterine cervix. In a study[2] a large proportion of patients were persuaded to test their own urine for sugar. Further studies are needed on the practicability of carrying out such checks on a large scale and on their possible effects on people's anxieties about ill health.

These three possibilities are not, of course, alternatives. Indeed, routine examinations by a general practitioner can be an opportunity for health education, and for dispelling anxiety and embarrassment.

Another way in which patients sometimes delay their own admission to hospital is by not accepting a bed when it is offered to them. Unfortunately systematic information about this was not collected, but some patients mentioned the point all the same.

'My husband had to go into hospital himself, so I asked them to put it off.'

[1] Backett, E. M., 'Future Role of the Family Doctor'.
[2] Mann, J. H., and Backett, E. M., Personal communication.

'I wanted my holidays, so I put it off.'

'I fixed the date to suit my business. I could have been in sooner.'

This sort of delay is less likely to be serious, since if it is important for the patient to go into hospital straight away, this can usually be explained to him.

Delays caused by the general practitioner

It has already been suggested that one reason for patients delaying consultation is their relationship with their doctor. Forty-five per cent of the general practitioners complained that some patients were too demanding and came to see them unnecessarily, for trivial complaints.[1] It is possible that, in trying to discourage patients of this kind from unnecessary consultation, the doctors may also discourage others or make these same 'demanding' patients hesitant about coming to see them with other, more serious, symptoms. It needs great skill to discourage only the unnecessary consultations and not all practitioners can be complete masters of this difficult art.

Once the patients did consult their general practitioner, what happened? Just over a third were referred to hospital at their first consultation. This is shown in Table 2.

TABLE 2

LENGTH OF TIME PATIENTS HAD CONSULTED GENERAL PRAC-
TITIONER ABOUT CONDITION BEFORE REFERRAL TO HOSPITAL
(Excluding maternity patients)

Length of time	%
Referred at first consultation	36
Less than a month	14
1 month < 6 months	14
6 months < 1 year	7
1 year < 5 years	18
5 years or more	11
Number of patients referred by general practitioner (= 100%)	512

The sign '<', which appears in some later tables as well as this one, means 'less than'. So '1 month < 6 months' means 1 month or more but less than 6 months.

[1] They were not asked about this directly, but they mentioned it spontaneously in reply to the question: 'Would you say you are satisfied or dissatisfied with the National Health Service conditions under which you treat your patients? In what way?'

Obviously the length of time people had consulted their doctor before being referred to hospital is not a measure of delay. During this time most patients were receiving treatment, and only when their condition did not respond, or deteriorated, was referral to hospital necessary. A relatively high proportion of the patients who had been under the doctor for a year or more had chronic conditions such as asthma, bronchitis, peptic ulcer and mental illness. For them this spell in hospital was but one episode in a lengthy illness. In addition, over a third of the people with a condition of the gall bladder had been under their general practitioner for a year before referral, nearly a third of those who had a prolapse operation, over a third of those with varicose veins or piles, and a fifth of those who had a hysterectomy or dilatation and curretage.

Only a small proportion of patients (4%) were directly critical of the general practitioner for not sending them to hospital 'as soon as it was necessary'.[1] Of course, these judgements should not necessarily be accepted at their face value. Patients may misunderstand or misrepresent what happened. Those who were chronically ill or whose illness was not alleviated by hospital treatment may have looked for an explanation or even for a 'scapegoat', and some may have cast their general practitioner in this role. Although there were so few patients who criticized their doctors in this way, it is worth while looking in some detail at what they said, first, in order to see whether there seems to be any substance in their criticism, and secondly, to see if anything can be learned from their experience.

Some implied that their doctor had made a wrong diagnosis.

The husband of one patient described how the general practitioner was treating his wife for 'a sort of nervous breakdown'. 'He gave her three or four different sorts of tablets, but she didn't get any better. She was losing strength and couldn't get out of bed without help. She kept going until around May, getting much weaker, then I said I'm going to tell the doctor I'm not satisfied. I said to him, "I'm not satisfied with the wife's progress. You must admit she's getting weaker not stronger. I want a specialist to visit." The specialist came and gave her a thorough examination—different to what her doctor had done. He looked up at me and said: "She should have been in hospital weeks ago. She's in a terrible way. Her heart's in a shocking state!" '

'He was treating me for about a month with laryngitis, I lost my temper in the end and he gave me a letter to go to the hospital. I thought I'd better do something about it. I'd been like it for weeks.' (Had lost his voice, admitted for nervous breakdown.)

'I think they were rather slack in dealing with the case on the whole. I wouldn't have had to suffer if he had done something. He kept saying it

[1] Question 9: 'Do you think the G.P. sent you to hospital as soon as it was necessary?' IF NO, 'Why do you feel that?'

17

was laryngitis—he's nearly 80. He shouldn't be on a doctor's list. Then I collapsed one day.' (Angina—had been consulting G.P. for last two years.)

Some were critical of the treatment he gave them.

'I have told my doctor frequently about the trouble and he just gave me bottles of stuff that didn't do any good. I insisted on going to hospital.' (Attended G.P. four years, admitted for pelvic floor repair.)

Others were critical simply of the delay.

'It seemed a long time before he did do anything. Three years is a long time to find things out. My periods stopped about three years ago. The doctor gave me tablets, but they had no effect. I thought the longer it was put off my chances got less—I don't know if that's right or not.' (Admitted for tests to find out reason for infertility. Since her spell in hospital this patient is arranging to adopt a child.)

A number felt their general practitioner was acting as a barrier between them and the hospital service, protecting the hospitals from too great a demand.

'Due to the shortage of hospital beds he put it off a bit. I think it's short-sighted.' (Bronchitis, bronchiectasis and emphysema developed pneumonia.)

'They don't like to crowd the specialist too much.' (Duodenal ulcer.)

And two illustrations from people who seemed to bear a grudge against their general practitioner were:

'My own doctor wouldn't send me to hospital; he said I was too far gone and didn't think anything could be done to help me.' (A man in his seventies with chronic bronchitis off and on for the last 20 years.)

'He didn't seem very interested. Said it was nothing to worry about, there were plenty of people worse off than you. He couldn't care less.' (Varicose veins.)

A further 1%, while not critical of the general practitioner who did refer them to hospital, described how they had consulted another doctor previously with unsatisfactory results.

'I'd been going to the other G.P. for about nine years. He treated me for thyroid, but when I changed doctors he took me off tablets right away and was interested in me and sent me to hospital for observation.' (Query tumour of ovaries.)

'I'd been going to the old G.P. four years. The new one sent me to hospital first time. Dr. —— wasn't really taking any notice of anyone at all. I must have had this diabetes five years and he hadn't found it out. But he could be forgiven a lot. He died while I was in hospital—had cancer all through his body.'

18

Finally, 2% had consulted their general practitioner about their illness, but had not been referred to hospital by him, and some of them were critical, either directly or by implication.

A woman in her sixties had been visited by her general practitioner at 8 p.m. He gave her some tablets and said, 'I'll see you in the morning.' She said, 'There's a nurse lives next door and she only came off duty at 11 p.m. and she phoned straight away for another doctor. He sent me away [to hospital]. He was very good seeing I wasn't his patient.' An operation at 3 a.m. revealed a perforated appendix.

A man who had been in hospital with pneumonia and a 'burst blood vessel' related, 'My doctor had died and in the interim there was a temporary doctor who wasn't interested. I fell on the icy pavement going to work on the 14th December. I went to the doctor on the 17th December and he said I had a touch of flu. I carried on till the following Tuesday, when I had to knock off work. I went to see the doctor on Wednesday morning with pains in the head. Christmas Eve the wife sent for him because I was semiconscious. He came and said, "He's on the turn." On Christmas Day, Sunday, the wife was worried and went for the doctor. His wife said he wasn't on. She—my wife—went to a policeman friend, who rang a doctor in H—— because the others were not available. The doctor came and said I had pneumonia. He said, "You'd better tell the other doctor he'd better be here first thing in the morning." Boxing Day he didn't come. My wife went to the policeman again, who phoned the doctor in H—— again, who said, "As far as I'm concerned it's a matter for the police." The policeman friend said, "You're talking to the police and I can't do anything without the doctor's sanction." (He had already phoned the Police Department, who told him that.) Within 15 minutes the ambulance was here—sent for by the H—— doctor. I'm not with that first doctor now—I wouldn't go to him. He's not a doctor; he's a vet.'

Apart from the patients who felt their general practitioner had delayed too long before sending them to hospital, for another 8% the initiative for referral had come from the patients themselves rather than the doctor—they had suggested it to him.[1] Just over half of these were maternity patients, and with only one—a woman having her fourth baby—had the doctor appeared to resist the suggestion.

'The doctor wanted me to have it at home. My husband wanted me to go into hospital this time, because he saw a bit of the third birth. I was a bit frightened at home when it was happening, at hospital I was more confident.'

The non-maternity patients who made this suggestion sometimes met opposition or indifference.

'The doctor tried to influence me against it—told me it would clear up,

[1] Question 10: 'Who first suggested you should go to hospital—you or the doctor?'

but I wouldn't be able to play the sports I want to.' (Operation on knee cartilage.)

'I asked him for a note. He never examined it.' (Piles.)

Some of these patients obviously felt that if they had not made the suggestion they would not have got into hospital as soon as they did, or perhaps even at all.

But these retrospective judgements may be erroneous. The fact that a patient is dissatisfied does not necessarily mean that there was unavoidable delay. Nor, on the other hand, does the fact that a patient makes no criticism necessarily mean that his admission to hospital was as prompt as it could or should have been. Clearly there will always be some conditions which are difficult to diagnose, but many patients will recognize this and be reluctant to criticize their doctor. Here are the stories and comments of two people who did not say that their doctor had delayed too long before sending them to hospital.

'I'd been to the doctor the week before for the first time, when I was three months pregnant. I told her I'd had a show and was worried. She said not to worry—lots of women have. Perhaps if she'd told me to rest, take it easy, not lift anything, but they don't sort of explain if there's anything wrong, so that you'd understand how things are. I had the miscarriage at home at five. The doctor gave my husband a letter to the hospital. My husband went with the letter and waited two hours, then we had to wait for the ambulance. I got in at eleven—it happened at five. I was lucky because I had a nurse stopping with me at the time.'

'It seemed a long time but in all fairness I suppose it was fair enough. I kept getting a pain in my side. The doctor said I'd probably have to have an operation, then he said it was probably an early change. This went on for six months, then I kept having such floodings the doctor thought it was the change and anaemia. The doctor said the best thing was to have the op. done and stop it. I'd been taking iron tablets for my blood. After they had finished the scrape they inserted radium. I didn't say anything, but when I knew about the radium I thought, "Oh I had cancer." '

In spite of the difficulty of interpreting patients' reactions, their views cannot be dismissed entirely. The great majority were satisfied with this aspect of their care, but it seems that for a small but significant proportion their admission to hospital was delayed by the failure of their general practitioner to make the right diagnosis at an earlier stage, or by his failure to recognize the severity of their condition. This is not so much a criticism of general practice as a recognition of human fallibility. One question which this raises is—should general practice be the sole channel by which most patients can reach the hospital service? At the moment virtually the only patients who do not come via their general practitioner are those who have accidents or who are taken ill suddenly. For the chronically or less dramatically ill, there is no other recognized means of approach. Of course, a patient can change his general practitioner—if there is another near enough—but to do this he must either explain to his doctor that he wants to change or wait for a fortnight after applying to the Executive Council, and he may be reluctant to do this at a time when he is ill.

It is difficult to envisage a satisfactory alternative approach to the hospitals, but since so much depends on the judgement of the individual doctor it is important to recognize that mistakes can be made and to provide safeguards for the patient. At the moment if a person's general practitioner makes an error of judgement it is difficult for it to be corrected. There are, indeed, three trends going on at the moment which may increase this problem. The growth of monopoly partnerships in small towns makes it more difficult for some patients to change their general practitioner. Where the work of the local authority maternity and child welfare clinics is being taken over by general practitioners, this removes the chance of another opinion for some patients. Finally, the discouragement of 'casuals' at departments meant for casualties eliminates the possibility of a direct approach to the hospital by the patient.

Is there, then, a need for another way in which patients could obtain a second opinion? This survey suggests that there may be.

Delays caused by the hospital

For people admitted to hospital directly as in-patients there was little delay, three-quarters going into hospital the same day as the general practitioner decided to refer them. But for those who were seen first at an out-patient department there were two possible periods of delay, first before they were seen there and then before they were admitted as in-patients. A third of the patients were seen at out-patients within a week of referral, another third in less than two weeks, 18% waited between two weeks and a month, 11% between one and two months, and 3% said they had to wait more than two months. The times between being seen at the out-patient department and being admitted were rather longer. They are shown in Table 3.

So 14% of the patients referred to out-patient departments at hospitals had to wait for a month or more before they were seen there, and 30% had to wait for two months or more between being seen at the out-patient department and being admitted to hospital. What did this mean for the people themselves? In many instances the delay was accepted without comment. Some people felt they had been relatively lucky. One who waited twelve months to have her varicose veins stripped thought 'it was very good, because loads of people have to wait about three years'. But some delays obviously lead to anxiety and distress.

A widow in her early sixties had had a hernia which had made walking difficult for her. 'I saw my doctor in July, but didn't see a specialist until August, and then there was no vacancy until January.' But, in fact, she had seen a doctor at a hospital two years previously in another area. 'He suggested it shouldn't be operated on until it was really necessary. When I moved here I hung on as long as I could, then when I couldn't go on any longer, I went to my own doctor.'

A man who had to wait five months before being admitted for his rheumatoid arthritis commented 'Well, I was bad, but there were only four beds in the hospital for this doctor. I was on drugs, cortisone, and then the leg broke out and they did something.'

A woman in her early forties with two teenage sons, related, 'When I went to see the specialist two years ago he put me on the waiting list to come in [for prolapse operation]. The hospital doctor said, "Try and carry on a bit longer." I don't think they ought to make you wait so long to get in.'

TABLE 3

TIME BETWEEN BEING SEEN AT OUT-PATIENTS AND BEING ADMITTED TO HOSPITAL
(Excluding maternity patients)

Length of time	%
Less than 1 week	20
1 week < 2 weeks	17
2 weeks < 1 month	17
1 month < 2 months	16
2 months < 3 months	11
3 months < 6 months	8
6 months < 1 year	7
1 year or more	4
Number of patients admitted from waiting list (= 100%)	319

Another patient waiting to have a prolapse repaired said, 'It was a worry wondering week after week if that letter would come.' Conditions for which at least half the patients had to wait two months or more for admission were varicose veins and piles (three-quarters waited that long), prolapse repairs, diseases of the bones and organs of movement, and diseases of the gall-bladder.

It is not possible, from the interviews with patients, to estimate the danger, discomfort, distress and temporary disability caused by these hospital delays. Some patients will always have to wait for a while, unless hospital facilities are increased so much that they are often underused. The problem is partly one of having enough beds for 'average' demand, and partly one of ensuring that patients in urgent need of treatment are seen and admitted straight away. The views of general practitioners give some indication of the implications of present shortages and delays.

Views of general practitioners on hospital delays

General practitioners were asked what they thought about the length of time their patients had to wait before they were seen at the hospital or before they were admitted. Altogether 74% of the general practitioners expressed concern on this score, and a further 23% said they sometimes had difficulties with certain groups of patients or types of illness. Half of them mentioned this problem spontaneously, before they were specifically asked about it.[1] Fifteen per cent were emphatically critical, using such phrases as 'ghastly', 'desperate', 'deplorable', 'hopeless'.

Many of the general practitioners described difficulties in getting old people admitted, although there was no indication from the sample of patients that old people had to wait particularly long. But our sample is, of course, confined to people who were eventually admitted to hospital and survived for some time afterwards. One general practitioner, commenting on the 'awful' difficulty of getting old people admitted said, 'You put them on the waiting list but they usually die first.' Another said that in his area hospital geriatric departments got in touch with the general practitioners when there was a vacant bed, as in so many cases the patient had died and they did not want to upset the relatives. Some comments of other general practitioners are given below.

'They're a big problem. They're the people we really can't get in. Unless something is done to create homes for them there is no answer. It's just lack of accommodation.'

'Geriatric admissions are always difficult. There's two years' wait, but I don't think it's any worse here than anywhere else.'

[1] Question 2: 'What do you feel about the relationship between general practitioners and hospitals in this particular area?' Question 3: 'Have you any suggestions about anything that could be done to improve the relationship in this particular area?' Question 4: 'What do you think about the length of time your patients have to wait before they are seen by the hospital—or before they are admitted?' Question 5: 'Are there any groups of patients—or types of cases—that you have particular difficulty in getting seen or admitted?'

'We obviously need an old people's home which is adequately staffed. You often have to keep people at home who ideally should be in oxygen tents. There were six or seven patients this winter I couldn't get in, with congestion of the lungs. If they're 75 or 80 I'd think, well we'll just have to manage at home. A lot more could be done for old people to make life worth living.'

The hospitals may be unaware of the extent of the demand as general practitioners become discouraged from referring old people.

'With old people—anybody I've tried to get in I've succeeded, but I don't very often try. I avoid trying, as there aren't any beds.'

Certainly, under the Hospital Plan[1] there will be a reduction rather than an increase in the number of beds available per 1,000 patients aged 65 and over. A number of the general practitioners complained that the hospitals did not consider the social difficulties.

'Hospitals allot priorities on the physical state of the individual, but forget the family background.'

'A medical emergency is O.K., but a social emergency waits until it dies.'

'The problem is the socio-medical emergency, the single elderly chronic sick person who struggles on helped by neighbours, the district nurse and the home help, who gets that bit worse, or the person next door who gets their dinner can't carry on any longer. It's a waste of time to try to get those into hospital—it take four months.'

One doctor explained how a patient of his, a woman of 79 with gross arthritis of the knee, had been seen at a hospital out-patient department and put in plaster. She had been taken home by ambulance, carried to her upstairs room, and left. She lived on her own and the lavatory, tap and coal were all in the yard downstairs. Fortunately the vicar had seen the ambulance and let the general practitioner know about it, and he arranged for her to go to a geriatric unit.

Several of the comments show that the difficulties general practitioners meet in making arrangements for elderly patients are not simply a problem of the hospital service, but are related to inadequacies in other institutional and in domiciliary services.

'With female geriatric cases you're often forced to admit them to a general ward; then they wait there a long time for a transfer.'

'Old people are very difficult when there's nobody to look after them. The welfare services are just on paper. In the country the home help service doesn't exist and now we have no district nurse. The old people's home is very good, but it just hasn't got places.'

Some old people could remain at home if they had domestic help, others could go into local authority homes if places were available. If neither of these are possible, the general practitioner may have to

[1] Ministry of Health, *A Hospital Plan for England and Wales.*

resort to getting the person into hospital.[1] These old people become victims of the division of our health and welfare services, being bandied round from one part of the service to another, a responsibility which each part is unwilling or unable to accept.

In one or two areas several general practitioners described appreciatively an arrangement whereby when old people were referred to the geriatric consultant he visited them and took over responsibility for admitting them or making arrangements for domestic help. Such an arrangement can co-ordinate the existing services, but when all types of facilities—home helps, hospital beds and other accommodation—are in short supply it can only alleviate some of the worst sufferings. Meanwhile, in areas where the services are not well co-ordinated some services are bound to be inefficiently used because other, more suitable, ones are not available.

Apart from old people, various other specialties were mentioned by a number of doctors as involving long waits, particularly gynaecology, orthopaedics and E.N.T. Sometimes the problem was one of balance: as one doctor put it—'Some waiting lists are enormous, others just days.' Others described particular circumstances which they regarded as unsatisfactory: 'Two months for an O.P. appointment for a suspected brain tumour.' 'Nine months' wait for a precancerous leukoplakia.' 'Six weeks before being seen when they may have cancer or may not—with vague symptoms which have to be investigated.' 'Medical cases not seen for six months—if you can keep the patient alive that long you don't need a consultant.' Indignation may lead them to exaggerate, and one patient who was seriously delayed is likely to be remembered by the doctor far longer than many who were admitted expeditiously. One doctor described how he had 'a patient with a chest pain—query coronary thrombosis. I referred him to out-patients in March and he was given an appointment in June. After this we were sent a letter to say the patient had failed to keep the appointment; in fact, he had died three weeks after the initial referral.' Others mentioned the working time people lost when they had to wait for operations. 'There's a big delay for orthopaedic operations. Sometimes a man will be off work three months, and six weeks he'll be waiting before an operation.' One said in a disgusted tone, 'There's three years' wait for hernia—in a working man!'[2] And another, 'Some hospitals give patients a truss until the operation, but it costs the country a lot of money'.

[1] See Forsyth, G., and Logan, R. F. L., *The Demand for Medical Care*. Horder, E., 'The Care of the Elderly'.

[2] See Carmichael, L., Ross, F., and Stevenson, J. S. K., 'Why Are They Waiting?: a Survey of Out-patient Referrals', for some more views of general practitioners on hospital delays, and some evidence on the time they wait before receiving a report of a consultation.

Many of the general practitioners suggested reasons or remedies for the delays and difficulties. There were a number of criticisms of junior hospital staff. One was that they were unhelpful about admitting patients.

'I had a baby born with an imperforate anus. The house surgeon said, "It doesn't sound very urgent to me." I had to go over his head.'

Another complaint was that they were reluctant to discharge patients.

'If they didn't do so many follow-ups, patients wouldn't have to wait so long.'

Elaborating this last point, the same general practitioner said that house officers tended to get patients to go back to out-patient departments every six weeks or six months, and, since the houseman himself was only at the hospital for a short while (usually six months), each one in turn was reluctant to discontinue the arrangement. This general practitioner went on to say, 'I was talking to a consultant the other day and I asked him why he didn't send patients back to us more often. He said some G.P.s would only send them back to hospital again. There's a hard core of G.P.s who just want to get rid of their patients.' This raises the general point of how the relationship between general practitioners and hospital staff affects the admission of patients.

The relationship between general practitioners and hospital staff

Their personal relationship with the hospital was stressed by several doctors as important in securing speedy admission for their patients. As one general practitioner put it: 'I have no problem. It depends on the individual doctor and his personal relationship with the hospital how well he can handle it'. Other comments were:

'It depends on your own status. The consultants here are my contemporaries. It might be difficult for a young man or a new-comer to the area. My patients don't wait. If they do I play hell with somebody.'

'Certain G.P.s are black-listed by the hospital, but we've got a good reputation as a firm.'

But when a general practitioner is 'black-listed', his patients are likely to suffer. One doctor was clearly on poor terms with the hospitals in his area. He showed letters from consultants saying: 'I protest most vigorously at you sending me a case you've not examined'; 'I don't see why this patient jumped the queue'; 'Please show a little more courtesy. I don't mind if you send me no more patients.' This doctor described how he had tried to get admission for a bed-ridden patient when the daughter-in-law who had been looking after her had a breakdown. He was told that the geriatrician would visit in a fortnight, but the patient died before that.

A number of patients described how their general practitioner had helped them get into hospital earlier than they would otherwise have done. For example, a man in his early sixties with a hernia was given an appointment at the out-patient department at one hospital for seven weeks later. 'I went back to my doctor and told him and he suggested cancelling the appointment and making me one at another hospital. He phoned the specialist there on Friday and I was in hospital on the Sunday. He (the general practitioner) was very good. That was a marvellous bit of work!' Other patients were more reluctant to approach their general practitioner.

A spinster of 50 had to wait 10 or 11 months for admission for a dilatation and curettage. 'I didn't pester him, but I was really at the end of my tether then. I should have been back to the doctor before—you've got to keep at them, everyone says.' But after she'd been put on the waiting list at the beginning of the year it was November before she'd seen her doctor again. 'He'd forgotten all about it. He's very forgetful. He rang the hospital that day. When he rang the specialist he apologized and said I'd been overlooked.'

Several general practitioners felt it was their job to see that their patients got into hospital as soon as necessary. 'It's up to the G.P. to make a bit of a fuss. If he feels it's too long he can ring up.' Others described the disadvantages of this system. 'If you push, you get a patient in earlier, but if you push too much you get unpopular.' 'In the old days a G.P. had a favourite consultant. Nowadays you accept that all consultants are good and get the earliest appointment. You find that the consultant you like everyone else likes and he has a waiting list of two months.' This general practitioner regretted the lack of personal contact that resulted from using different consultants —'As it is, you know them as names rather than as people. If I used the same one he would accept my word in relation to investigation and would know I had a bee in my bonnet about certain things.' This shows how a doctor's desire to reduce the time his patients have to wait sometimes conflicts with his wish to develop personal relationships with individual consultants.

Avoiding delay: private and domiciliary consultation

One way in which some doctors helped their patients to avoid long waits was by referring them to a consultant privately.

'They often have to wait a very long time before they are seen at outpatients with skins. I tend to advise patients to see a consultant privately.'

'My chief complaint is the long waiting list for O.P. appointments—so

27

much so that patients say "Could I see the man privately?" They're prepared to pay so they can be seen earlier.'

'For paediatrics there's a long wait for out-patient appointments. A lot go privately. There was one girl—I found a murmur and there would have been a long delay, but she went privately. The consultant found a coarctation of the aorta. If she hadn't had an operation soon, it would have been fatal—I wasn't expecting that.'

Another doctor said—'If you want a case seen urgently it can be seen privately tomorrow, but a farm labourer waits. Money talks still.'

Three per cent of the patients in our sample had consulted a specialist privately before admission and a similar proportion (not all the same patients) went into hospital as private patients. One of the main reasons they gave for seeking private advice or treatment was to avoid delay. But if some patients 'jump the queue' in this way, the effect may be to make others wait longer than they would have done if there was no private practice. And while this system exists there will be the suspicion that part-time consultants have a vested interest in maintaining a waiting list so that some patients will consult them privately. Public pressure to reduce delays is also likely to be less as long as they can be avoided by patients who might otherwise be influential in demanding improvements in the normal Health Service.

Private medical care might be regarded as an alternative route to the hospital for patients who are dissatisfied with the action prescribed by their general practitioner. But, in fact, it is most frequently used to avoid delays at the hospital when the need for hospital care is already recognized by the general practitioner. Only one patient in the sample had consulted a specialist privately because she was dissatisfied with her general practitioner. The other people who consulted specialists privately did so for administrative reasons, to avoid delay rather than clarify diagnosis. One reason why private consultation is not an effective route to hospital for patients whose need is not recognized by their own general practitioner is that few people know how to get it without the help of their doctor. In any case, medical etiquette discourages private consultation with a specialist without a letter from the patient's own doctor.

Another way to speed up admission is by domiciliary consultation. A quarter of the general practitioners said spontaneously that domiciliary consultations were useful for this purpose, another 15% said this when they were asked directly.[1] It is possible that others felt the same, but were diffident about saying so. One went so far as to say:

[1] Question 13: 'What do you feel about domiciliary consultations?' Question 14: 'In what way do you find them most useful? Do you ever use them for getting patients admitted?'

'They're used by certain consultants as a form of blackmail—and I'm prepared to sign that. You ring up for an appointment and find the first appointment is in two months unless you have a domiciliary consultation.'

Some of the others who had found them useful in this way felt that they were a method of making the consultant appreciate the patient's difficulties at home. 'If you can't convince the house surgeon the patient needs admission, the consultant can find a bed when he's seen the patient at home.'

But some general practitioners had found that the consultant preferred to admit the patient rather than visit him in his home.

'In some cases when you ask for a consultant to visit he says send the patient in—when you've already been refused admission.'

'A consultant who doesn't do them causes unnecessary admissions. I had a patient at home recently with malignant hypertension. I asked the consultant to do a domiciliary, but this consultant doesn't do them in this area, he said, "Send the patient in." This was unnecessary, as nothing could be done; the main aim was to reassure the relatives.'

When some consultants are too busy to do domiciliary consultations, one way to decrease the demand for hospital beds might be to increase the number of consultant posts.

Altogether 7% of the general practitioners were critical because some consultants were unwilling to do domiciliary visits. At the same time three mentioned specific instances which they felt were abuses of the system. One said:

'I had a patient who obviously had to be admitted. I rang the registrar, who agreed to admit her. He rang me next day and said the consultant would do a domiciliary. I said no, I would get her admitted elsewhere.'

But the majority of general practitioners, 63%, were enthusiastic about this form of contact with the hospital service. Although at least two-fifths sometimes found them useful for getting patients admitted, this is not necessarily an abuse of the system, but rather a useful 'safety valve' in an organization which might otherwise become too rigid.

Summary

In looking at the three possible sources of delay in getting to hospital—the patient himself, his general practitioner, and the hospital—information from the patients suggests that they themselves are the most frequent, if not the most serious, impediment. About a fifth felt that they had delayed too long before consulting their doctor. Their reasons were often vague, but ignorance, fear, embarrassment and unwillingness to bother the doctor were the ones most frequently given.

29

A small proportion of patients, 5%, thought that their general practitioner had not sent them to hospital soon enough and, while one should not necessarily accept their judgement, the stories they relate, and also some of the stories told by patients who did not make this criticism, suggest that for a few their own doctor acted as a barrier between them and the hospital care they needed.

Once patients were referred to hospital, two-thirds were seen at the out-patient department within a fortnight, and 70% were admitted within two months of being seen there. But some had a much longer wait, and evidence from the general practitioners suggests that the effects of hospital delays are occasionally serious.

General practitioners are in many ways better able to evaluate the importance of delays than the patients themselves, and they are also very much aware of the problems of patients who are not admitted because of inadequate facilities. It is therefore disturbing that so many of them were forthrightly critical about the delays and difficulties in getting patients seen and admitted. The importance they attach to this suggests that more should be done to reduce delays and increase the number of beds, in particular for old people. But present plans are for relatively fewer beds for old people in the future.

What can be done to reduce delays? Education of the public and changes in the relationship between patients and general practitioners may encourage people to seek medical advice as soon as they are aware of certain symptoms. Changing patterns of disease and medical treatment suggest that general practitioners might usefully turn their attention to the detection of disease at the pre-symptomatic stage. Some of the delays which arise through misjudgements by general practitioners might be avoided if patients realized it was not unreasonable to ask for a second opinion.

The major source of delay appears to be inadequate facilities, or inefficient use of present resources by the hospital service. This, at any rate, is the view of many general practitioners. Because of these deficiencies they refer some patients to private specialists, but the continued existence of private practice probably aggravates the general problem, although it reduces the delay for some. Other possible improvements are a closer relationship between hospital staff and general practitioners, so that each is more aware of the other's problems; and more consultants available for domiciliary consultation, so that patients are not admitted unnecessarily. But the greatest need is probably for more money to be spent on beds and services for old people. One general practitioner put it this way: 'The delays are unfortunate but unavoidable in the circumstances. The Government won't spend the money.'

PART TWO

Life in the Ward

III

NURSES AND WARD ROUTINE

WHAT is it like to leave your home and family and go into hospital, where you are dependent on strangers for physical care and companionship? Of course, the answer varies, depending on what is wrong with you, what sort of hospital it is, what sort of person you are and so on. Some of these variations are discussed in the last part of the book. This chapter and the next two are about three important influences on the day-to-day life in the ward—the nurses, the other patients, and the size of ward.

Nurses work[1] and patients live in the ward. The way they get on together can promote comfort and relaxation or anxiety and frustration. Much depends therefore on the skill and sympathy of the nurses, and it should be borne in mind that two-fifths of the whole-time nursing staff in hospitals are either student nurses or pupil nurses.[2]

Patients' views of nurses

Some idea of patients' views of the nurses and other hospital staff is given by their answers to the question: 'What struck you most about your experience in hospital?' which was asked right at the beginning of the interview. Two-fifths were entirely enthusiastic and the most frequent subject for praise was 'the hospital staff', 'everybody'. As many as a third of the patients made such comments as: 'They couldn't have been better to the Queen'; 'I think they are very kind and do their best for you'. Another quarter specifically praised the nursing staff, a tenth the doctors, and one in seven the personal atmosphere, using such phrases as friendly, kind, cheerful or happy.

---

[1] One study showed that nurses spend a third of their time 'at the bedside'. Willcock, H. D., *Nursing Methods in a General Hospital.*

[2] Ministry of Health, *Report for the Year 1961, Part I: The Health and Welfare Services.*

Altogether two-thirds made some favourable comment about the people in hospital or the personal atmosphere. The other items mentioned favourably with any frequency were the food, by 22%; the physical surroundings, by 10%; and their medical treatment, by 5%. Just under a fifth of the sample were mainly critical. The doctors or the nurses were criticized by 11%, while 8% commented that the hospital was understaffed. Six per cent were critical of the food and similar proportions of the physical conditions, the other patients and early wakening. Four per cent mentioned noise, 3% restrictions and regulations, and another 3% their medical treatment. So, looking back on their hospital experience, it was the people they met who made the most vivid impression, and they spoke about the nurses more frequently than the doctors.

When asked to describe the way the nurses (and midwives) looked after them,[1] just over half, 53%, of the patients were unreservedly enthusiastic—'like angels', 'real champion'. Only 3% were mainly critical at this stage, but when asked if there was any occasion when they felt the nurses could have done more for them, and for examples of occasions when a nurse was particularly kind or unkind, nearly a quarter, 23%, made some critical comment and another 15% some qualification which did not amount to a criticism.[2]

Much of the praise was in very general terms—kind, nice, pleasant, looked after us very well. A fifth of the patients commented on how much the nurses did for them—'nothing was too much trouble', 'they'd do anything for you', 'they made a fuss of you'. A tenth described the nurses as cheerful, friendly, jolly, homely or talkative; 7% said they were hardworking, 4% described them as efficient or well trained, 3% as thoughtful, patient, considerate, sympathetic or understanding, 1% as strict, and a similar proportion as skilful or gentle. Other descriptions were: 'They had hearts of gold and nerves of iron', 'You didn't feel embarrassed with them at all; they did things naturally'.

The examples patients gave of occasions on which a nurse or midwife had been particularly kind were often of extra things that the nurses had done for them like posting letters, shopping, washing and setting their hair, or washing a nightdress. Some forms of attention which might be generally considered part of routine nursing care evoked gratitude apparently because they were often of such an

[1] Question 45: 'Can we talk about the nurses (and midwives)—how would you describe the way they looked after you?'
[2] Question 46: 'Was there any occasion when you felt they could have done more for you?' Question 47: 'Can you give me an example of an occasion when you thought a nurse (or midwife) was particularly kind?' Question 48: 'Was there any occasion when a nurse (or midwife) was not very kind—either to you or to any other patient?'

intimate character. 'They used to wash you and help you like that, keep you nice and clean.' 'They did not mind taking me to the lavatory.' Even patients who did not seem to have had very good nursing care expressed appreciation of the attention they did receive. 'They never let you lie in bed more than a week before they gave you massaging so you didn't get sore.'

Several other stories they told were about the nurses' sympathy and understanding.

'Well, there was one night—I suppose it comes to everybody. About the second night I became homesick and I began to snivel and cry to myself like. I thought nobody would hear, but a nurse came up and said, "What's the matter dear?" I said, "I can't help it, but I'm homesick", and she bent down and put her arms right round me and gave me quite a hug and said, "Don't worry, everyone gets like that. We all feel like that. Now go to sleep and you'll feel better in the morning." And I did. Now, wasn't that kind?'

One man put it this way. 'We're not sentimental, but when you're ill a little kind word is worth a lot of bullion.'

Among the minority of patients who criticized the nurses a number described occasions when the nurses were felt to be unkind, impatient, inconsiderate or unsympathetic.

'One nurse was nasty. I heard her slap a girl once because she was making a row over her first baby. She wasn't married and the nurse made a show of her before all the other patients.'

Some of these criticisms were about the nurses' treatment of old people.

'The night nurse wasn't very kind; there was one old lady who was a cripple and when she rang the bell for attention the nurse was cross and irritated with her.'

'An elderly man was moaning; they told him to be quiet. I felt it very much. He was so ill.'

A few patients felt they had not got the right medical treatment.

'They said the bandages should be changed every day, but they didn't always do them. You don't like asking really, because of them doing so much.'

'I was on tablets every four hours, but sometimes there were six hours between one lot and two between the next. You had to take them at the same time as other patients were due, to save trouble.'

Others described what they felt was inadequate nursing care.

'Mrs. ——, she's dead now, she had no control over her water. She ought to have been changed more often. They just left her lying there. I felt terrible.'

Another occasional complaint was that some nurses were unskilful, untrained, or not gentle.

'Some, because of lack of experience, are a bit clumsy, but most of them were very careful. Some just shovelled the food in and you choked. The night nurse was not very gentle with the injection.'

Several described occasions when they or other patients had not been able to get a bed-pan or bottle.

'There was one man there who'd had a leg amputated because of gangrene and he used to call for a bed-pan and several times they didn't come. Sister said he could hold himself. Then he did it in the bed. He said, "It's not my fault, it's not my fault." I think it used to worry him. One occasion I got out of bed and told a nurse and she said she had only got one pair of hands, but she was only washing bottles at the time. The nurses didn't put themselves out.'

'One lady, she'd had a stroke, and she kept calling for a bed-pan and they ignored her. That was the only thing I'd got against them.'

There were a few complaints that nurses were authoritarian. 'You're just treated sometimes, well, like delinquents, as though you're stupid. They're not actually unkind; they just treat you like a child.' 'There's always the odd one or two who treat you like naughty children.' Only one mentioned an overprotective attitude—'They want to help you all the time; I'd sooner get up myself.'

Many of the patients who were at all critical qualified their criticism by some explanation for the nurse's action. Several of those who described incidents when nurses had been sharp or impatient justified this by criticizing the patients.

'The nurse will lose her temper occasionally and then take it out on a patient, but it's usually the patient's fault.'

'If the nurses were sharp with any of the young mothers—well, I think they deserved it. You don't go in to be pampered, but to have your baby and get well again.'

'You can't expect nurses to stand by and get belted by mental cases. It's only right that they should belt back'.

Others excused the nurses' thoughtlessness or lack of skill because of their youthfulness, referring to them as 'teenagers' or 'only young bits of lasses'.

'Some of the nurses are very young. It's hard for them to take things seriously. The older ones understand better. The other patients used to complain they were always laughing, but I never worried.'

'The trouble with the nurses is that they are too young to be doing hospital work. Eighteen is too young. They are a bit irresponsible. They were a bit hopeless except at routine nursing.'

But the most frequent explanation for the nurses' shortcomings was that they were overworked.

Understaffing

A quarter of the patients who were at all critical of the nurses said spontaneously that they thought the hospital was understaffed,[1] and 13% of all patients said this.

'They would have done more for you if they'd had the time.'

'They have too much to do; they get harassed.'

'You never actually saw a nurse for hours. They couldn't do more for you, because there weren't enough nurses. The girls didn't have enough time to do things. They didn't have enough patience with one old gentleman who kept messing the bed. They hadn't enough time to attend to him.'

Obviously if hospitals are understaffed[2] this is likely to affect both the physical comfort of patients and their sense of ease and security. As one put it: 'They were shockingly overworked and you naturally suffered as far as the attention went. That's not a criticism of the staff, but they couldn't cope.'

A few patients instanced occasions when, presumably because of the shortage of staff, they had been asked by the nurses or other patients to do jobs which they did not feel were appropriate.

'What I objected to was two-night nurses; they used to shout in the morning, "Who's going to light the fire for the tea?" '

'As long as some of the patients who were knocking around would empty urine bottles the nurses would let them. Not that they told them to. If you were walking the length of the ward someone would be sure to ask you to empty the bottle. And I'm one of those people who can't do that sort of thing, and I was rather embarrassed when I had to refuse. I don't think that sort of thing should go on at all.'

'One nurse gave me clean sheets to put on my bed and I was supposed to be resting, and on the day after I came in the staff nurse appeared with the elevenses on a trolley and said, "Here you are, Mrs. Simpson, get on with handing out the elevenses." Well, I was shocked, downright shocked, but I said to myself it's a matter of two things: I either refuse

[1] Question 2: 'What struck you most about your experience in hospital?' Question 18: 'Do you think the accommodation and provision for patients could be improved in any way?'

[2] Rather surprisingly, national figures on the number of unfilled nursing vacancies are not available; the Sheffield Regional Hospital Board Nursing Committee found the following deficiencies in March 1962: trained nurses and midwives 19·7%, enrolled nurses 25·7%, student nurses 34·9%, and pupil nurses 36·4% (*Hospital and Social Service Journal*). As the deficiencies for student and pupil nurses were greater than those for trained and enrolled ones, the position seems more likely to deteriorate than to improve.

to do it and tell them I'm in for a rest or I get up and do it and then drop on the floor, and I nearly did. I don't know how I lifted the teapot. I did murmur a bit of a complaint and the nurse said sharply, "We are here to tend the sick and the dying, not to make tea for the patients." The only helpers were volunteer helpers who were grateful ex-patients. Even one paying patient washed the pots with me one night. Two bad heart cases came back and served teas every day. I suppose they were duty bound.'

These comments show how a shortage of ward orderlies or ward maids may affect patients' relationships with nurses, and aggravate feelings about inadequate attention. One or two patients felt that nurses had to do inappropriate jobs.[1]

'I don't think nurses should dust—a ward maid should do that.'

'The thing that struck me most was first and foremost the lack of domestic help. The nurses had so many duties including so much cleaning that I felt the patients did not have sufficient attention.'

Unfortunately it is not possible in this study to relate patients' views of the nurses to the extent of staff shortage in the different hospitals or wards. Although patients often explained nurses' shortcomings by saying they were overworked, it is possible that this was just the most acceptable explanation from the patients' point of view. To be dependent on nurses who were unsympathetic or unreliable might have been so distressing that some patients felt impelled to look for other, more impersonal, reasons for their perceived neglect. On the other hand, some who were critical of their nursing care may not have looked beyond the immediate cause of their displeasure. When they wanted attention they may not have been aware of other demands on the nurses' time. So, while some patients may have imagined that nurses were understaffed when they were not, others may not have realized that their nurses were overworked. Whether or not overwork or understaffing was the main reason, to a minority of patients their nurses appeared too preoccupied or harassed to give them the attention they would have liked. And it is not only the amount and type of work the nurses did which influenced patients' attitudes towards them, but also the way in which the work was organized.

The ward routine

Patients who were awakened early proved to be more critical of the nurses than those who were awakened later, although no patients

---

[1] Willcock found that nurses in the hospital he studied spent an average of 8% of their working time doing domestic work and a further 11% preparing and clearing meals or preparing and giving beverages. Op. cit., p. 13—Work assignment Unit.

Nurses and Ward Routine

mentioned this directly as a reason for feeling critical of the nurses. The proportion expressing some criticism of the nurses was 40% among those wakened before 5 a.m.; 25% between five and six; and 17% at 6 a.m. or later.[1] Not unexpectedly, many of those who were awakened before 5 a.m. felt this was too early.[2] This is shown in Table 4.

TABLE 4

TIME OF WAKENING AND PATIENTS' OPINIONS

Time	Patients woken at that time		Proportion who found it too early
	Number	%	
Before 5 a.m.	50	7	74%
5 a.m.<5.30 a.m.	203	28	68%
5.30 a.m.<6 a.m.	196	27	45%
6 a.m.<6.30 a.m.	187	26	24%
6.30 a.m.<7 a.m.	50	7	17%
7 a.m. or later	37	5	0%
All times	723	100	44%

If patients were not woken until 7 a.m. it seems as if there would be virtually no criticism on this score, but in fact 95% of the patients in our sample were woken before this, while 62% were woken before 6 a.m. and 35% before 5.30 a.m. Only two patients felt the time was too late.

A number of the comments the patients made about the early wakening show their readiness to see the nurses' point of view. Two who were woken between 6 and 6.15 and described this as 'all right' said, 'They had their work to do', 'The night staff have to get around to it before the day staff come on'. Another two who were awakened between 5.30 and 5.45 and thought this too early qualified this by saying, 'I've often thought it could be altered, but the night nurses have so much to do and they're understaffed', 'But they've got to do that to get the work done'. Some replies reflect people's adaptability and acceptance of strange habits in a different environment: 'I didn't sleep very well. You got a cup of tea at quarter past five, which was nice. I don't think it's too early. After all, the nurses have got to get

[1] There is a similar pattern when maternity patients are excluded.
[2] Question 20: 'What time were you woken up in the morning?' Question 21: 'Did you find that too early, too late or about right?'

on with their work. I used to be glad to get up then and shave and then I used to go back to bed and sleep until breakfast.' But other comments illustrate the way in which early waking causes irritation with the nurses. One patient who was awakened before 5.15 said:

'You're tired by the time you've had breakfast, but they don't like you going back to bed, because you make the beds untidy. I feel, with all due consideration, that surely the patients are more important than tidiness.'

This not only voices dissatisfaction with the hospital routine, but questions the values on which certain regulations are based. Apart from being wakened early in the morning, a number of patients described how it was difficult to get enough rest in hospital.

'I think they disturb the patients too much, coming round making the beds. You're just getting comfortable and they came round and make you uncomfortable.'

Irritation with bed-making was expressed by a number of patients, and it is clear from their comments that this also can be a source of friction between nurses and patients.

'There's all this flapping about getting the beds straight. You mustn't lie on top of it; you must be in it, not on it. Before matron's round the auxiliary was in a panic and said, "Please either get off the bed and sit in a chair or take off your dressing-gown and get into bed." You mustn't leave the dressing-gown on the bed. In the army all this regimentation would be called "bull".'

'They were dressing the beds up every half-hour. They put you in like sausage meat and bind you down so that when matron comes everything is beautiful. They're at the beds every flipping minute.'

This shows, too, how the relationship between nurses and patients can be influenced by the discipline imposed on the nurses by their seniors. The ward sister is a key person here. Under the matron, and with day-to-day instructions from the medical staff, she has responsibility for nursing the patients, for the management of her ward, and, if the hospital is a training school for nurses, for arranging the practical instruction of the students.

Patients' views of the sister

When they were asked to describe the way the ward sister looked after them, 63% were entirely enthusiastic and 4% mainly critical, while the remainder were less extreme.[1] The most frequent specific praise of the ward sister was that she was efficient—12% said this, 7%

[1] Question 51: 'What about the ward sister—how would you describe the way she looked after you?'

described her as strict, 6% as approachable, friendly or understanding and 10% said they had little contact with her. So her ability to 'do her job' was mentioned by twice as many patients as her sympathetic attitude, and in a number of instances patients seemed to feel that the first precluded the second.

'She was very efficient, but rather cold. You didn't feel she gave individual attention like the nurses did.'

'She was very efficient and she knew her job, I grant you, but she could have been more human to the patients. You just couldn't talk to her right. You didn't get to her. You couldn't confide in her or speak to her if you were in trouble.'

Some sisters apparently managed to combine both attributes.

'She was lovely. She had such a grip on the ward you could see her word was law, but with the patients she was just ordinary and easy.'

'She was charming, most efficient and nice. She had a most wonderful way of approaching the patients.'

Some of the comments of those who were enthusiastic suggest that they regarded the sister as someone apart.

'She was a toff—very, very nice.'

'She was inclined to be strict, but dedicated you know. But she was beautiful, like a nun. We all loved her.'

'That's a lady, from her toes up. She was a lovely girl.'

Others seemed to have had a warmer relationship with her.

'She looked after us very well. She was very sporty. We had a sweep on the horses.'

'There were two there, very nice. You could talk to them; they weren't standoffish.'

Most of the few criticisms were of a sister's authoritarian attitude.

'She was too strict. She carried everything a bit too far. She had no time for you, but you felt she knew what she was doing.'

'She rather liked treating us like naughty children.'

'She was more officious than efficient.'

The most forthright criticism of all described the ward sister as 'the most cruel person I've ever met. She ignored us. She wasn't human—she was hard and callous.'

The sister has in many ways an unenviable position, between nurses, patients and doctors. Sometimes she may 'identify' herself more particularly with one of these groups, and this may affect her relationship with the others. Some of the patients, for instance, when they were asked about how they thought the nurses got on with the sister, suggested that her concern for the patients made her somewhat unsympathetic towards the nurses.

'She was a bit harsh with the nurses, but I've never heard her talk harshly to a patient. The nurses respected her, but they were frightened of her.'

'She was wonderful, really wonderful. She had all her patients' interests at heart. But I tell you one thing, when sister's off the nurses do get a bit slack. Mind you, she was a proper disciplinarian. They didn't get on awfully well, because she was so strict. She'd been 42 years on that ward.'

'She looked after you well, but she wasn't liked by the nurses. She was too dogmatic. She did show several of them up, which I felt quite unnecessary. It made us all feel uncomfortable.'

Others felt the sister was too lenient with the nurses, and that the patients suffered in consequence.

'She was very pleasant, but not very efficient, not much discipline. The nurses seemed to get on quite well with her, because she just let them do as they pleased. I sometimes think the old battle-axes are better from the patients' point of view—they make sure the nurses are doing their job.'

'She was all right, but I don't think she was quite strict enough—too easy-going.'

Thus, while several patients described her as strict, others felt she was not strict enough. But many sisters seemed to have resolved this possible conflict and appeared, at any rate to the patients, to get on well with both patients and nurses.

'She was very good. She knew her job and how to do it. Some sisters are so stiff and starchy with their juniors, but here they worked hand in glove.'

'She was a good sister. She wasn't a bully and knew her work. She kept the nurses in their place, but they all spoke well of her. One of the nurses said you could always ask her questions; she'd never make fun of you and say you ought to know that.'

Altogether 15% of the patients felt that the relationship between the sisters and the nurses was rather unfriendly, half the patients felt they had a good relationship with each other, and the remainder that it was satisfactory.[1]

Comments reflect how pleasant relationships create a happy atmosphere which is appreciated by the patients.

[1] Question 52: 'How do you think the nurses (and midwives) got on with the ward sister?'

42

'They got on very well. The whole attitude of the ward was cheerfulness. It was a happy ward.'

'They got on fine. She got a good name from the nurses. They liked to be on that ward.'

Revans,[1] studying 15 hospitals, found positive associations between the extent to which ward sisters have confidence in their seniors and in hospital organization, and 'the extent to which the sisters see it as their responsibility to help in the integration of student nurses'. It seems likely that the perception the nurses have of those in authority over them, whether one of co-operation or of hostility, will be transmitted to the patients they are looking after.

Data from our survey show that patients who were critical of the sister were four times as likely to be critical of the nurses as those who described the way the sister looked after them in enthusiastic terms. (Table 5.)

TABLE 5

PATIENTS' VIEWS OF THE SISTER AND OF THE NURSES

	Views of Sister*		
Views of nurses*	*Entirely enthusiastic*	*Intermediate*	*Some criticism*
	%	%	%
Entirely enthusiastic	63	38	27
Intermediate	22	34	13
Some criticism	15	28	60
Number of patients (=100%)	463	159	48

* These two attitudes are not directly comparable, as different questions were asked about nurses and the sister.

Such an association would arise because some patients were generally enthusiastic and others generally critical, and this may be part of the explanation here. But it is probable that ward sisters who have good relationships with their patients encourage their nurses in the same way.

There are obviously other ways in which nurses' satisfaction with their work is likely to affect patient-nurse relationships. For example, Revans[2] has suggested that the average length of patients' stay is

[1] Revans, R. W., 'Hospital Attitudes and Communications'.
[2] Revans, R. W. ibid.

Life in the Ward

lower in hospitals where morale is high. From the patient's point of view, then, it seems relevant to consider the general level of satisfaction within the nursing profession.

Satisfaction in the nursing profession

Some information about this is available from other studies. In 1947, the Working Party on the Recruitment and Training of Nurses found that just over half the student nurses did not successfully complete their training. Studying the reasons for this loss, it is suggested that the first significance was in hospital discipline and the second the attitude of senior staff. No comprehensive study has been carried out since then, but various regional inquiries suggest that the wastage has not greatly declined. Barr,[1] studying student nurses who joined four general hospital training schools in the Oxford region during 1951–3 found a third were unsuccessful. Cross and Hall[2] in their survey of entrants to nurse training schools in the Birmingham area found a wastage of 59% and concluded that 'the overall bed availability could increase by 6% if sufficient staff were available'. Wright[3] found the wastage rate among Scottish student nurses in 1957 was similar to that in the 1947 Working Party report for general hospitals. In all these later inquiries the unsuitability of the entrants emerged as the main reason for wastage. And another study in East Anglia[4] suggested that 'standards for acceptance are being lowered in an effort to meet the demand for more nurses in the hospital service'.

But whether the main reason for the wastage rates is the educational unsuitability of the applicants or the 'type of discipline that pervades the training schools',[5] such high rates suggest that many nurses who are doing their training are dissatisfied or uncertain of passing their exams. Their sense of strain may sometimes be communicated to patients. One who criticized a nurse for her authoritarian attitude related how this nurse had said, 'If I don't pass this time I'll go and get a job in Woolworth's.' The patient commented that she would have been better there.

Studies by the Nuffield Provincial Hospitals Trust[6] have criticized the 'traditional' system of nursing and 'the custom of organizing the work as a series of jobs, or parts of jobs, each to be done by a different

[1] Barr, A., 'Training of Student Nurses'.
[2] Cross, K. W., and Hall, D. L. A., 'Survey of Entrants to Nurse Training Schools and of Student-nurse Wastage in the Birmingham Region'.
[3] Wright, M. S., *A Study of the Characteristics of Successful and Unsuccessful Student Nurses in Scotland.*
[4] 'Student Nurse Wastage, East Anglia', *Nursing Times.*
[5] Working Party on the Recruitment and Training of Nurses *Report*, op. cit.
[6] Nuffield Provincial Hospitals Trust, *The Work of Nurses in Hospital Wards* and *Studies in the Functions and Design of Hospitals.*

nurse proceeding from patient to patient round the ward. This gives the patient a service which is to some extent both unsatisfactory and unsatisfying—unsatisfactory because responsibility for the attention given him is arbitrarily divided between several people, unsatisfying because the attention itself is apt to be impersonal.' They conclude 'that there is little time available to the nurse to enable her to establish human contacts with patients and relatives'.

The Oxford Area Nurse Training Committee, in a study of student nurses,[1] found that 'the student nurses mentioned the lack of time in which to carry out procedures as the feature of the ward situation with which they were least satisfied. In many wards the student nurses found it difficult to distinguish any direct chain of command . . . (and) they felt there was a general lack of meaningful relations with other people in the hospital.'

These various studies all suggest that student nurses, at any rate, are often working under conditions of stress which are likely to decrease their efficiency. This in turn is likely to affect both the physical care that patients receive and the sympathy and understanding the nurses give them.

Summary and conclusions

Most patients were grateful for the way the nurses had looked after them. Dissatisfaction among the minority may have stemmed from three sources: unreasonably critical or demanding patients; individual nurses who were unsympathetic or otherwise inadequate; and unsatisfactory working conditions for the nurses. It is not possible to distinguish between these possible reasons for discontent.

In the next chapter it will be seen that nearly half of the patients felt that *other* patients were sometimes too demanding. On the other hand, at least a third of the examples they gave of occasions on which they felt nurses were unkind related to their treatment—or neglect—of other patients, not themselves, so not all the critical comment can be dismissed as arising from self-centred, over-demanding patients.

Any profession is bound to attract some unsuitable recruits, but this is possibly more serious in the nursing than in most other professions, since so much of the day-to-day nursing of patients is done by nurses who are training. Other studies have shown that between about a third and a half of nurses do not complete their training, mainly because they prove to be inadequate academically. Critical comments from a minority of patients suggest that a few may be unsuitable for their exacting job because they are unsympathetic or

[1] Oxford Area Nurse Training Committee, *From Student to Nurse.*

have been inadequately trained in the skills of human relationships. As nursing becomes more highly developed greater technical skills will be needed, and it is probable that greater emphasis will, and should, be put on technical and academic competence in the selection of nurses for full training. At the same time, nurses need careful training and supervision in these skills of human relationships; otherwise we may have more specialized and highly skilled nurses providing more impersonal and less sympathetic care.

Several patients described the difficulties under which they felt the nurses worked. Understaffing or overwork were mentioned spontaneously by one patient in eight and by a quarter of those who were at all critical of the nurses. National figures are not available, but in some areas at least there is a shortage of nurses, and patients are likely to feel that they suffer as a result of this. The organization of the nurses' work in the ward also led to occasional friction between nurses and patients. Early wakening and frequent bedmaking were two things that were apt to irritate patients. From the nurses' point of view other studies have revealed a low level of satisfaction among some student nurses, and this, too, is likely to affect the way patients are looked after.

In spite of these difficulties, over half the patients described the way the nurses looked after them enthusiastically. This is a tribute to the devotion of most nurses. The criticisms voiced by other patients suggest that the hospital service, and the community as a whole, may be placing too great a strain and counting too much on this selfless devotion.

IV

PATIENTS AND PRIVACY

WHILE nurses look after patients' physical needs, and can encourage confidence or allay anxieties, they are often too busy and preoccupied to spend a great deal of time talking to patients. It is on their fellow patients that most people rely for companionship.

When asked who they talked to most while they were in hospital, four-fifths said they had talked more to the other patients than to the nurses, doctors or their visitors.[1] Just over half, 53%, had talked to other patients 'a great deal', 32% 'quite a bit', 11% 'not very much' and 4% not at all.[2] But, as a number remarked, 'In hospital you can't choose your own company.' Some felt they had been lucky in their companions.

'I talked to everybody and got on very well with the chap in the next bed. I think the sister has a lot to do with it, in choosing where she puts you. I think possibly this one did consider whether we would get on with the chap in the next bed.'

Others were not so satisfied.

'It depends on the other people. Some of them are very snooty. If one of the girls hasn't got an ultra-modern dressing-gown and slippers they look down on her.'

'Some patients should have been in another hospital. One or two were queer and wee'd on the floor. They were beyond conversing with.'

Nevertheless, in spite of the fact that patients cannot choose their companions, most of them, 61%, said they had found their contacts

---

[1] Question 76: 'Who did you talk to most while you were in hospital—your visitors, the doctors, the nurses, the other patients—or anyone else?'

[2] Question 77: '(What about the other patients) did you talk to them a great deal, quite a bit, or not very much?' Two-thirds of those who had not talked to other patients at all were in single rooms.

with other patients 'very enjoyable'; 34% described them as 'fairly enjoyable' and only 5% as 'not very enjoyable'.[1]

Patients who had appreciated the company of others described how they had played darts, dominoes, billiards and cards together, and had run sweepstakes. Sometimes they sounded as if they were describing a holiday camp rather than a hospital.

'They make you feel at home. The night before I came out we had a sing-song and a strawberry tea and a game of lexicon. And there was one woman had her birthday and they brought a cake and put it in front of her while she was asleep. Then they woke her up singing "Happy birth-day to you". It makes a difference, you know.'

'We talked for hours on end—a perfectly happy fortnight. The outside world doesn't matter any more. You get frightfully nosy about everyone inside.'

A number commented that contact with the other patients had helped 'to pass the time' and relieve boredom and loneliness.

'We used to go in all different wards and make friends. It was the only bit of pleasure you used to get.'

'It was a bit of company. You're lonely in hospital.'

Several mentioned the interest they had derived from conversations with people they would not normally have come into contact with.

'Some patients are quite interesting—talking about their lives and hobbies. One man was a pigeon man. He told us about it. I learnt something.'

'There's a friendliness in hospital you don't get elsewhere—no class distinction.'

'You get to know other people's lives—see the other side of life.'

Some described the help they had given other patients by making drinks and taking plates round. 'More often than not I used to make the tea of a morning, so I had more of a chance of talking to the patients.' Others referred to the support that they had given each other.

'We kept each other going. They were very considerate just after I'd had the operation. Very friendly.'

'The chap in the next bed had the same trouble. We were commiserating. Then congratulating each other when it was all over.'

Patients' discussions together about their illnesses and treatment are described in more detail in a later chapter. Sixty per cent found

[1] Question 78: 'On the whole did you find these discussions very enjoyable, fairly enjoyable or not very enjoyable?' The 4% who did not talk to other patients at all have been excluded.

the discussions helpful and few, 9%, upsetting.[1] Several patients described the reassurance, encouragement and confidence they obtained from these conversations. Others stressed their own satisfaction in helping and reassuring others.

'The woman in the next bed was frightened. I told her she needn't be frightened. I wasn't. You used to forget your troubles when you were talking and it made you feel at home.'

'The patients boost up each other's morale. There was one fellow who was a bit depressed. I heard him in the hymn singing, he had a voice like a crow. I went up to him and said, "That's a fine baritone voice you've got"—his voice was terrible. It lifted him up; from then on you heard him all the time.'

Some had been interested in the conditions and treatment of others.

'At one time I would have thought it dreadful to have a breast off—but one lady there had and she got on fine.'

'They do enlighten you, don't they? You get to know about things; you never realize so much is done when you've not been in these places.'

'I was in with three caesareans. It's an experience you hope will never happen to you, but it's a sharing.'

A sense of comradeship was described by some people who had clearly found it helpful to 'get things off their chest'.

'Everyone was quite thrilled to have given birth to a child. It gives you more confidence if you discuss anything.'

'You relieve your own mind talking about yourself. It takes a bit of the strain off.'

'I found out that other people were going through the same thing and I didn't feel so lonely.'

One who had been mentally ill said, 'You find that they have experienced the business that people were shunning you. We talked about it and its mental effects.' And one who had had a stillbirth commented, 'I used to get edgy at first when people talked to me about it, but I got better. There are some things you don't like to talk about to your parents and it was nice to talk about things.'

A few had been comforted by the reflection that others were worse than they were.

'You found there were people a lot worse off than yourself and they came up smiling at the end of it.'

'You think you've got a lot, but someone else has got a damn sight more, worse than you. You think yourself lucky.'

[1] Question 79: 'Did you discuss your illnesses or treatment together a lot, a little or not at all?' IF A LOT OR A LITTLE, 'Did you find these discussions at all upsetting—sometimes or generally? Did you find them at all helpful?'

Life in the Ward

There are many ways in which the companionship of other patients can support and cheer patients during their stay in hospital. But there are others aspects of this intimate companionship with strangers who are also ill which are less pleasant and helpful.

Distress and anxiety

A substantial minority of patients, a quarter, found the illnesses of other patients worrying or distressing.[1] When a patient dies, this is clearly depressing for the other patients. The event is not only distressing in itself; it casts a gloom over the ward, and can awaken patients' fear of death for themselves. In this century, and in our urban society with small families, death has become an increasingly unfamiliar event and a subject generally regarded as unmentionable. To be close to someone when they die is obviously an upsetting experience, and in hospital patients' apprehensions and anxieties about their own health may be heightened by their illness and separation from home.

> 'I used to hear in the morning that that old lady had died and this old lady had died. I used to wonder if I'd ever get out of there.'

> 'Especially when they were dying, we rarely had a day pass without somebody pass out. They used to move them up to sister's end. I hoped they wouldn't move me up there.'

Although removal to a side ward may alleviate some of the distress, it does not dispel it all, and, of course, it may increase the apprehension of the patient who is moved.

> 'There were one or two bad cases. Three died. One shouted for three days. They put her in a side ward and she got quieter then. It was a bit upsetting, though.'

When casualties are brought in and die this may cause even more disturbance and distress than the death of chronic patients.

> 'There should be a special place for bad car crashes—the victims. There was one brought in about 12 and she died about 3.30 and it upset everyone. We all knew, you see.'

And even when the death does not occur on the ward, patients may learn about it and find concealment more fearful than disclosure.

> 'There was an 18-year-old girl who didn't come out of the anaesthetic. They told us on the ward that she had moved to another part of the hospital. I don't think those things should be kept in the dark. I think it would be better to be told.'

[1] Question 81: 'Did any of the illnesses of the other patients or the treatment they were having worry or depress you at all?'

50

Patients and Privacy

It was not only people dying that distressed patients. Old people sometimes caused anxiety. Some patients were upset by the treatment the old people had received.

'The old lady—nobody seemed to come near her—not even the doctors. We felt sorry for her and it depressed us. Perhaps there wasn't much they could do for her—I don't know.'

'They were taking in old people that nobody else would take, and the poor dears were always needing bed-pans and the nurses just pushed by them, because they hadn't time to deal with them. It was very upsetting. Some of the old people had been taken in just to relieve the family situation and they weren't cared for much.'

Others had been disturbed by old people who were mentally ill.

'Some of the old people used to talk a lot in their sleep. There was one who used to scream out at night and used to talk all sorts of rubbish like "The house is on fire".'

'A casualty came in at night and she kept shouting for the Vicar and said she saw fairies and elephants and her sister standing by the bed. It frightened me. I thought she would come and bang against me. My husband spoke to the sister and she moved her away from me. She was 70 and lived alone and had been in a fire in her home.'

There were those who were upset by the immediate after-effects of other patients' operations.

'I used to be depressed on operating day seeing the other patients come back from the theatre. It was worse for those who were going to have the same operation.'

'I dreaded watching them come back from the theatre and come round —they were usually sick.'

'I don't think they should bring patients back to the ward until they have come round from the op. Then they could come round decently in a side ward.'

And some who were made anxious by the preliminaries to operations and the patients' absence from the ward.

'I didn't like watching people got ready for operations. They went down for a bath, then they were put in a white shroud and laid out in a mackintosh.'

'It upset me when the ops. went down to the theatre. It's because I'm nervous. I worried about them until they came back.'

The frequency with which patients with cancer were mentioned as a cause of distress possibly reflects the widespread fear of this disease. The validity of the diagnosis may well be questioned in some

51

instances, but once the 'diagnosis' has been made it seems to lead to a feeling of awe and concern which may be unrelated to the realities of the situation.

'There was a chap who said he had fibrositis and did nothing but moan all day. I found out afterwards he had cancer, so it changed my attitude.'

'One woman had cancer in the womb and was having radium needles. She was only 38. I felt for her.'

'I felt depressed about a chap opposite. He was suffering from cancer or gangrene. He got worse—he went from a robust man to a weak one. It gets on a person's mind, watching one like that. I think he should have been put in a single ward.'

Then there were patients with conditions which were unpleasant to look at.

'One person had a thyroid op. and, as I thought I was going to have one, I was upset, because she was going round with no wrapping or anything over her neck and I hated to see it. As it happened, I didn't have a thyroid op., but I won't ever go and have it done now I have seen what they did to her.'

'There was one woman who'd had her breast removed and you could see all this terrible stuff draining into her bottle under her bed. I'll never drink Oxo again.'

'There was just one girl, she was 14, and she was covered in eczema. I would never go in the bath straight after her. Mind you, she was a nice girl. They told us it wasn't catching.'

And then there were others who had been upset in a variety of ways:

'There were a few cases of glaucoma. It destroys the sight. I felt I might be getting it—a patient told me the symptoms. It preyed on my mind.'

'There was one—just a piece of marble that couldn't move. They were sending her out, because they couldn't do anything for her.'

'The only thing I didn't like was when they were actually giving birth to their children in the ward and some of the girls cry and call for their mothers.'

Irritation and embarrassment

Distress and anxiety about other patients' illnesses were not the only reason people had for wishing some patients had not been in the ward with them. Altogether 29% of the patients wished this, and over half of these said they had not been worried or depressed by the illnesses of other patients.[1] (Table 6.)

[1] Question 80: 'Were there any patients you wished were not in your ward? Why was that?'

TABLE 6

ATTITUDE TO OTHER PATIENTS IN WARD AND TO THE
ILLNESSES OF OTHER PATIENTS

(Excluding patients in single wards)

	Wishing other patients were not in their ward	
Found illnesses of other patients worrying or depressing	*Yes*	*No*
	%	%
Yes	43	17
No	57	83
Number of patients (=100%)	199	497

Some described patients who they felt were dirty, who swore, or who had very different standards from themselves.

'He was a disgusting fellow with a low mentality and he was ignorant. He was 67 and he would get out of bed and expose his private parts to the patients. He was very indiscreet and would never put his pyjama pants on and would bend down purposely and do his water on the floor without waiting.'

'There was only one fellow and he'd cough over you at the dining-table. I was all against that. I was in a real state. You never know what you can pick up off a fellow like that.'

'There was one girl, she was dirty and she didn't have a maternity bra. Oh, she was a pest; she used to come cadging fags and she didn't have any visitors and after we'd had ours she'd cry and get nasty. And one time when her baby cried in the night she kicked the cot and shouted, "Shut your fucking mouth." She'd had two babies and didn't know the father of either of them.'

Several people described how they had been disturbed at night by other patients. 'There was one lady who was in dreadful pain during the night and when I lay awake I heard her moaning.' 'One man who was 81 years old was a bloody nuisance, but you could excuse him really on account of his age. He was shouting day and night for bed-pans. Towards the end sister moved him so we could all have a good night's sleep.' 'We had one, during the night she would get out of bed and clip clop down the ward in wooden mules. I would have thrown her out of the window cheerfully.'

A few related how there had been arguments or disputes over the television or radiogram.

'One chap there was rather a grumpy bloke. He wanted the record player turned off—started shouting, "I'm ill." He might have been a big shot outside, but he was just one of a crowd in there. But we had to turn the record player off—it had been lent to us by a doctor for Christmas.'

'There was a young girl, she was only 18 and she was a diabetic. I felt sorry for her, but she would have her own transistor set on loud and there were times when I could have picked her up and thrown her out of the window. But I suppose she was allowed it to cheer her up.'

Then there were the ones who were talkative:

'She told the same story over and over again to every patient who came in. We used to feel like winding her up. You wouldn't think anyone had ever had a baby but her.'

And the ones who grumbled:

'There was "Mona Lott". She was always discussing her family from one end to the other. She neither read a paper or knitted.'

Some complained that other patients expected too much of the nurses:

'One of them I wished to hell and back. She wouldn't do anything to help herself—wanted nurses all the time.'

When they were asked directly about this, nearly half, 47%, felt there had been some patients who were too demanding.[1] Most of the comments were fairly general.

'Some thought they were in a first-class hotel. They expected too much of the nurses.'

'Very ungrateful some of them were. In fact, one or two of the patients were inclined to treat the nurses as though they were servants.'

'Some people, they'd grumble if they were to be hanged; they'd want a new rope.'

'There were several like that. You'd think they'd had their bloody head off.'

There was some criticism of people who were felt to be snobbish.

'There was one woman, she was just that little bit above us, you know, her husband was something in the college. They used to bring the bed-pans round after meals, but she never wanted it when it was there; always waited that little bit afterwards and then called nurse.'

[1] Question 82: 'Do you think some of the patients were too demanding? In what way—can you give me an example?'

'The bloke in the next bed, an old major in the Army, he thought he'd bought that ward. A nurse was never allowed to pass that bed without he wanted something. He was a nasty piece of work.'

Many of the comments again turned on bed-pans and bottles.

'There were times when fellows kept on asking for bottles. When the nurses were really busy they sometimes had to wait. Some of them seem as if they won't help themselves.'

'There was one person, she thought she ought to have all the attention. She wouldn't go to the toilet and she wouldn't have the bed-pan. They had to bring the chair down.'

Some of the widespread feeling that other patients were too demanding may have arisen because of inadequate staffing or other facilities in the hospital.

'One fellow had asthma and wanted oxygen. Well he can't get it all the time—others want it, old fellows usually. This fellow was 80; you can't fight old age.'

When nurses are very busy and a ward is understaffed this is likely to give rise to a feeling of competitiveness among the patients for the nurses' attention, and this will make them critical of each other's demands. As some patients put it:

'You get a few that likes a little fussing and on the other hand some don't get it at all that need it.'

'Those who make the most noise get the most attention, while others didn't perhaps get as much attention as they ought to have had because of the demands of other people. The person who tries to be a model patient tends to get pushed into the background.'

While irritation with other patients can be aggravated by staff shortages, embarrassment with some of their habits is accentuated by inadequate privacy, and this of course can also make patients feel embarrassed on their own account.

Lack of privacy[1]

Thirteen per cent of the patients felt that they did not get enough privacy.[2] A few made general comments about this.

'You never feel you have enough privacy in hospital. It's just a matter of embarrassment. Some people don't have any and that's all right, but if you haven't got that hardness you feel it more.'

---

[1] The 33 patients, 4%, in single wards have been excluded from this section.
[2] Question 72: 'Did you feel you have enough privacy?' IF NO, 'In what way?'

'I don't think you really get privacy. For the first one you feel as if you've lost all your modesty. After that you think—well, we're all here for the same thing.' (Maternity patient.)

Most of those who complained described a particular aspect of this lack of privacy. For some it was not being able to see their visitors without being overheard or seen.

'You couldn't talk about anything private with your visitors. It would have looked funny to ask for the screens.'

'They don't pull the curtains when you have visitors, everyone can hear what you are talking about. We've got past the sloppy stage now, but I did feel sorry for the young couples with their first baby.'

Others referred to the fact that they could not discuss things with the doctor privately.

'I suppose that's always a thing you have to get used to in hospital. When the surgeons and that come round all the patients can hear what he's saying.'

'During the examination everyone can hear what you're asking. I think it would be nice if they took you into a private room off the ward.'

A number said that the lavatory doors could not be locked and others mentioned the washing and bathing arrangements.

'I think the bathroom business was the worst. You can't lock the doors in hospital. There was a notice on the door, but you can imagine how much notice some men take of that. It really wasn't very pleasant.'

'There wasn't any privacy at all unless somebody was really ill. There was only one bathroom and they never shut the door. I'm rather sensitive about that sort of thing.'

Several people complained of what happened when patients had to use bed-pans.

'There were no curtains in the ward. You had bed-pans in front of everybody.'

'I used to be shy about them putting you on a bed-pan with no screens. You may be all women together but you've got your bit of modesty.'

'When you wanted the bed-pan they used to bring the screens round, but there was always the odd gaping hole and they could see you.'

'The sister would come in with a pile of bed-pans. "One for you, one for you", and say, "Right girls, get ready for swabbing." No screens or anything, it was really very embarrassing.'

And there were various other ways in which patients complained of a lack of privacy.

'When your husband came up and little personal things you like to do to yourself, like when I used to make up because I haven't any colour. They used to pass remarks. They were older and used a bit themselves, but they didn't like to see younger people using it.'

'I wished they would draw the curtains when you get out of bed into a chair. After an op. the wind gets locked in your tummy. You don't want everybody to see your face then.'

'I wanted to have a good cry when I'd had Kenneth and I thought if only they'd draw the blinds. I felt if I had a good cry it might relieve me, but I didn't want anyone to see me like that.'

'When I wanted to use the bed-pan I felt they heard me; if I made a bigger noise everybody would hear when I was on it.'

Several of the comments referred to the curtains and screens.

'There is no privacy in hospital; You couldn't pull your curtains round you when you wanted.'

'You had screens round you, but you didn't feel private.'

Altogether 57% of the patients were in wards that had curtains which could be drawn round their beds, 40% had a movable screen, 1% had cubicles, and 2% said there were neither curtains nor screens, but a third of this last group were in two-bedded wards. The proportion who felt they did not have enough privacy was greater in wards with screens than in wards with curtains, 16% compared with 10%. Comments from two of the few patients with neither screens nor curtains were:

'You had to undress in front of everybody. You were exposed to everybody. We would have liked something, but we didn't have screens or curtains, and we're not young girls any more.'

'All that was done to you was in full view of everyone—treatment and everything.'

Ten per cent of the patients in wards with screens or curtains felt that the screens or curtains were not always used when they would have liked them to be.[1] This proportion was also higher in wards with screens than in wards with curtains, 13% compared with 8%, which is not unexpected, since moving screens is likely to involve more effort for the nurses than pulling curtains. Some of the patients made comments about these methods.

[1] Question 74: 'Were there any occasions when they did not draw the curtains/move screen round you and you would have liked them to? When was that?' Question 75: 'What about the screens/curtains round the other patients—were there any occasions when they were not drawn and you would have liked them to be?'

'I should have liked the screens round a little more often, but the nurses were busy and I didn't like to ask.'

'The screens are a disadvantage. I like the curtains—they're a great asset. When they run out of screens it's just too bad.'

'The screens want some pulling round. They never refuse you, but you've got to wait your opportunity to get someone to do it for you.'

'Curtains are not all that satisfactory, they tend not to be drawn properly or they get pushed around while you're dressing at the side of the bed. Perhaps they could have Marley folding doors in lightweight plastic material, and it would be easier to clean, too.'

But failure to use the curtains and screens does not account for all the feelings of inadequate privacy. Just under half the 13% who had complained that they did not have enough privacy felt that the screens or curtains were not used enough, and 5% of the other patients also said this, so altogether 18% felt there was some lack of privacy in one form or another.

Patients may be embarrassed or distressed either because the curtains or screens are not put round them or because they are not put round other patients, and, in fact, these two complaints were made with equal frequency, 3% saying they were not always drawn round themselves, and 3% round other patients, while 4% made both complaints.

Some of the comments of people who thought that the curtains were not always drawn round them when they would have liked it were:

'They didn't leave the screens round me when I had the tube up my nose and I was just an exhibition.'

'Sometimes they weren't too particular. I had to have injections for two or three days—on my backside. I imagine some of the other patients would have wished they'd drawn them round me.'

'One day when the doctor and 10 students came to see me they couldn't all get in the curtains so they left them open for all the ward to see and hear.'

The other occasions when they would have liked them drawn, apart from the often-repeated 'when you're on the bed-pan', were for shaving (female), swab taking, treatment, bed-baths and for feeding babies.

Some of the occasions on which they would have liked screens or curtains put round other patients are cited below.

'On weepy patients. If they were screened off you would *feel* they weren't so near you and they wouldn't get you down.'

Patients and Privacy

'One day we had a lady who was dying and when they treated her they didn't draw the curtains at all, and when you're not feeling very well yourself it's not too nice, is it? You could see them put in the tubes from down below for passing her water and tubes down her nose for feeding.'

'The old people used to soil the bed and it wasn't very nice to see them change the linen and wash them. Also two of them passed away and they didn't put screens round until the very end. There were young girls in there too, 9 and 12 years old, looking on and feeling frightened.'

'There were two cancer patients—they had tubes in their mouths and down their throats. Another one started to vomit the minute food came round. It was very rare that the curtains were drawn round. I just couldn't eat—as soon as I started I felt it would choke me. I did tell one of the nurses, but it didn't make any difference.'

TABLE 7

ATTITUDES TO PRIVACY—MEN AND WOMEN PATIENTS
(Excluding patients in single wards)

	Men	Women	
		Non-maternity	Maternity
	%	%	%
Type of Ward			
With curtains	48	63	59
With screens	48	35	39
Other/nothing	4	2	2
Not enough privacy	7%	15%	22%
Curtains/screens not used enough*	4%	12%	19%
Number of patients (= 100%)	267	331	107

* Those with neither curtains nor screens have been excluded.

Women were more likely than men to be in wards with curtains, but in spite of this they more often complained that they did not have enough privacy (Table 7). Maternity patients were the ones most likely to make this complaint, and this is probably related to arrangements for feeding babies. Some mothers had commented on this.

'When I couldn't feed the baby they were all watching to see what happened that time. I think it would have been better on my own.'

'When I was having difficulty with feeding with the breast pump and all that and all the other girls were having to watch.'

'One of the patient's husbands came in once when I was feeding him and they didn't put the screens round.'

Again women were much more likely to complain that the curtains and screens were not used enough. Fourteen per cent said this, compared with only 4% of the men, although in general it has been shown that this complaint was made more frequently in wards with screens than in wards with curtains. It seems probable that nurses are more punctilious about this in men's wards, and comments from some of the women patients suggest that some nurses may feel that privacy is less important in a female ward.

'I'd have liked the curtains drawn when I was using the bed-pan and getting washed. They used to say "You're all women", but I like my privacy.'

'Sometimes when you were feeding the baby there were men walking past the door and they could see in. We got a screen and put it by the door, but the nurses used to come and shift it.'

So far the discussion has been concerned with the minority of patients, just under a fifth, who said they had felt some lack of privacy. Only a few of the others made any comments about this aspect of their hospital care. Some were appreciative of the privacy they had.

'They were so careful about the curtains. I was sitting watching television in the ward when the anaesthetist came to see me. He took me back to my bed and pulled the curtains round just to tell me that the next day he would give me an anaesthetic.'

'They were grand about that—when they were dressing wounds and all that. If they didn't the sister scotched them up about it.'

Other comments suggest that they had not been wholly satisfied, but were not prepared to be definitely critical.

'The patient in the next bed was asked about things which revealed she had had a baby before she was married. I feel it would have been better if she had been asked about this before she went into the ward.'

'In a public ward you could not expect any more. Some fellows are inclined to be a nuisance, but that isn't the fault of the hospital.'

One positively rebuked us for asking a question he felt was frivolous or irrelevant. 'You go into hospital to get better. You don't go in to have a good time or to have privacy.' Another considered the disadvantages of more complete privacy. 'You can't really have more (privacy) unless it was private. I wouldn't like that; you'd have no contact with the other patients.' This last comment introduces the problem to be discussed in the next chapter—the size of ward.

Summary and conclusions

Altogether two-thirds of the patients described some disadvantage of being in a ward with other patients, and a rather similar proportion described some advantage.[1] These two views were unrelated in the sense that the proportion expressing appreciation of some aspect of their contact was similar among those who did and those who did not describe some disadvantage. Half the patients were critical of some aspect of their contact while appreciating others.

Thus, most people both appreciate some aspects of their contact with other patients, and are distressed and embarrassed by others. The problem is therefore not one of deciding which patients appreciate privacy more than company. Most, if not all, want both. Some people in certain circumstances have a much stronger preference for one than the other, but in general the problem is to maximize the advantages of companionship and minimize the disadvantages.

There are one or two obvious ways in which the disadvantages can be reduced. Curtains seem to afford greater privacy than screens and are likely to be more used. They are also less demanding of the nurses' time and effort. But although they may cut out certain distressing or embarrassing sights, and so create some sense of privacy, they do not cut out sounds and smells. In this inquiry no specific questions were asked about noise, but other studies[2] have shown that patients are the main source of disturbance, and naturally it is at night that most irritation is caused. If there were more single or side wards for new admissions, seriously ill and disturbed patients, this would reduce the disturbance and enable other patients to have more peace and rest.

More complete privacy than that afforded by either screens or curtains seems to be needed for much treatment if other patients are not going to be worried and distressed by observing it, and the patients themselves are to be protected against the inevitable, usually well-intentioned, but occasionally embarrassing, curiosity of others.

---

[1] Disadvantages were lack of privacy, illnesses of other patients which were worrying or depressing, patients they wished were not in their ward, patients who were too demanding, and discussions about illnesses which were upsetting. Advantages were enjoyable discussions with other patients and discussions about illnesses which were helpful.

[2] Dewar, R., and Sommer, R. 'Disturbing Noise in a Mental Hospital'; Statham, C., 'Noise and the Patient in Hospital'; and Hayward, S. C., Jefford, R. E., MacGregor, R. B. K., Stevenson, K., and Wooding Jones, G. D. E., 'The Patient's View of the Hospital.'

Again, this could be achieved, to some extent, by the use of treatment rooms for dressings and so on, and recovery rooms for people who have had operations. There is also the point that screens and curtains do not provide adequate privacy for consultation. Suitable occasions and places for doctors and patients to talk in private need to be provided.

Although there are various measures—more curtains and side wards, recovery rooms and the greater use of wheel-chairs to take people to the lavatory—that could be achieved with relatively minor modifications in existing hospitals, they may be regarded as palliatives, alleviating some of the distress caused by the presence of other patients without creating a real sense of privacy. In new hospitals should more radical experiments be tried, so that many more patients have rooms of their own? Some evidence about patients' reactions to wards of different sizes is given in the next chapter.

V

WARD SIZE

THE last chapter showed how lack of privacy affected relationships between patients. This chapter shows how the size of ward influences patients' attitudes both to each other and to the nurses. It starts by discussing what size of ward patients were in, and what size they said they preferred.

Four per cent of patients were in a room of their own, and 12% in rooms with two, three or four beds. At the other end of the scale, 41% were in wards with at least 20 beds and 13% in ones with 30 or more. When they were asked whether they would have preferred a room of their own, a larger or smaller ward or a ward the same size,[1] three-quarters of all the patients said they preferred the size of ward they were in and 8% that they would have liked a single room. The association between their preferences and actual size of ward is shown in Table 8.

These figures need to be interpreted with care, since people's experience of wards of different sizes is likely to be limited and this expressed preference may merely reflect their adaptability and general willingness to make the best of things. Because of this limitation, the proportion preferring the size of ward they actually were in may be a useful statistic comparatively, but before definite conclusions can be drawn for hospital planning, controlled experiments are needed inside hospitals.

Bearing this limitation in mind, these figures suggest that ward sizes of five to fourteen beds may be most popular. Three times as many people would have preferred a smaller ward as those who wanted a larger ward, and among the small group who wanted a larger ward one-third had been in single rooms and half in rooms with one or two beds. The proportion preferring the size of ward they were in was lowest for single rooms, comparatively low for larger wards

[1] Question 71: 'Would you have preferred a room of your own, a smaller ward, a larger ward or a ward the same size?'

with 25 or more beds, and highest, over 80%, for wards with five to fourteen beds.

TABLE 8

PREFERENCE FOR WARDS OF DIFFERENT SIZES

	Number of beds in ward									All patients
	1	2, 3	4	5–9	10–14	15–19	20–24	25–29	30+	
Prefer:	%	%	%	%	%	%	%	%	%	%
Ward same size		78	70	84	83	75	73	69	65	74*
Room of own	57									
		6	15	7	3	8	5	4	2	6
Smaller ward	—	—	5	4	11	13	15	25	30	13
Larger ward	29	10	5	4	2	4	2	—	—	4
Uncertain ...	14	6	5	1	1	—	5	2	3	3
Number of patients (= 100%)	28	48	40	109	119	84	149	48	94	719

* Those in a single room who preferred it, 2% of all patients, have been included here.

Relationship with other patients

The predominant reason they gave for liking the ward they were in or wanting a larger ward was that they appreciated the company of other patients. Here are some of their comments:

'I'd sooner be among the others. You help one another to get better. The well patients help the nurses and can go and chat to the sick patients.' (Ward of 20–24.)

'I prefer a big ward. I like a bit of company. Time passes quickly. It's a little bit of comfort seeing other people get better and go out having had the same operation.' (Large ward—number of beds not known.)

A number of those in large wards with 20 or more beds described the friendly atmosphere there and explained the advantage of size in establishing good relations between patients.

'In a single room you get bored, but in a ward that size you get to know everybody, but you don't see enough of them to get sick of them.' (Ward of 20–24.)

'I prefer a large ward, because you pass the time of day with one another. In a small ward perhaps there's someone very sick, so you can't have a joke.' (Ward of 20–24.)

'I like a large ward. You can have a few more laughs. A small ward can be depressing if people are miserable. A large ward is a source of interest—you can watch everybody.' (Ward of 30 or more.)

But some of the people in large wards would have preferred a smaller one because they felt it would have a more intimate atmosphere.

'In a smaller ward you can mix more with the patients. In a big ward you can't talk to everybody.'

'You set up a little group, say five beds on each side, and when you totter around you find the people up the other end are strangers. Only those within hailing distance are friends.'

Others in wards with less than 10 beds felt that the smallness of the ward had contributed to their feeling of comradeship.

'It was very nice—six beds. It was a small community. I'd detest to be on my own.'

'You get to know the people better. It's quieter.' (5–9 beds.)

'It's just nice, that size of ward. I think in very large wards, well, if you're ill in bed you can only nod to people over the other side. I think you get terribly bored. But in a little ward you can all talk together.' (5–9 beds.)

TABLE 9

SIZE OF WARD AND ATTITUDES TO OTHER PATIENTS

	Number of beds in ward							
	2 or 3	4	5–9	10–14	15–19	20–24	25–29	30 or over
Found illness of some patients worrying or depressing	11%	22%	21%	23%	22%	26%	38%	33%
Wished some patients were not in their ward ..	17%	20%	21%	27%	37%	35%	29%	31%
Thought some patients were too demanding	27%	30%	38%	38%	49%	56%	56%	66%
Number of patients* (= 100%) ..	48	40	110	119	85	130	48	94

* People who gave inadequate answers have been excluded when the percentages were calculated.

In fact, enjoyment of the companionship of other patients turned out to be unrelated to the size of ward, when patients in single rooms were excluded. But worries and irritation with other patients increased with the size of ward, as can be seen from Table 9.

The proportion who found the illnesses of some patients worrying or depressing was three times as great in wards with 25 or more beds as in small wards with two or three beds, and the proportion who wished some patients were not in their ward was also less in small wards than in large ones. One obvious reason for these differences is that the chance of an ill or irritating patient being in the same ward is directly related to the number of patients in the ward. As one patient said:

'I prefer a ward of four to six. If you're in a small ward, there's less chance of anyone dying or anything tragic like that happening in your ward.'

Nursing care

Several patients felt that they either got or would have got more attention in a small ward.

'They were small, nice little wards. You get more attention in a small ward. There's too much for the nurses if it's bigger.' (Ward of 10–14 beds.)

'With a small ward they've got more patience and time. With a bigger ward they haven't time to bother with everyone.' (In ward with 10–14 beds, would prefer smaller one.)

'Twenty-four's too many, if all the beds are full. The nurses can't cope with it all.'

Not every patient shared this point of view.

'I'm not fussy, but if anyone is really ill I think it's an advantage to be in a big ward. I'll give you an example. A patient about four beds away from me took a seizure and within one minute he was being attended to. The ward is so big the nurses are always there. The ward is never empty. With all of us there we spotted him and the nurses whipped up and got the oxygen going.' (Ward of 30 or more beds.)

The proportion of patients who felt that some of the other patients were too demanding rose, as Table 9 shows, from 27% of those in wards with two or three beds to 66% of those in large wards of 30 or more. Feelings of competition for the care that is available are likely to increase with the size of ward, and with it the anxiety that they may get less attention because of the demands of other patients.

Table 10 seems to support this. It suggests that patients in large wards with 25 or more beds were more critical of the nurses than those in smaller wards, while those in single rooms, or wards of between four and 14 beds were the most enthusiastic about their nursing care.

TABLE 10

SIZE OF WARD AND ATTITUDE TO NURSES
(Excluding maternity patients)*

Attitude to nurses	Number of beds in ward								
	1	2, 3	4	5–9	10–14	15–19	20–24	25–29	30 or over
	%	%	%	%	%	%	%	%	%
Entirely enthusiastic	70	50	73	61	63	46	54	46	51
Intermediate	17	34	10	16	23	36	28	26	22
Some criticism	13	16	17	23	14	18	18	28	27
Number of patients (= 100%) ..	23	38	29	77	94	72	141	47	90

* Maternity patients have been excluded, since they were likely to confound the analysis. They tend to be in small wards and to be relatively critical of the nurses.

Attitude to single rooms

While large wards were slightly less popular than others for several reasons, many patients were emphatic about not wanting a room of their own.

'I was offered a room on my own, but I didn't want it. I like company. If you're on your own, you think too much. I wanted something to take my mind off it.'

'I wouldn't want a room of my own. I had one once. You're imprisoned. You have to press the bell and you don't know if the nurse hears it.'

'I shouldn't want to be on my own. I'd go mad with only four walls to talk to. If I had a lot of money I wouldn't go into a private ward. I might pay for more attention, but no matter what your standard of living or class you need company. Even the people from private wards were glad to come in for a chat.'

Although nearly a third of the patients in single rooms said they would have preferred to be in a ward with other people, there were still more people who would have liked a room of their own than there were single rooms available, 57 against 33, but, of course, not all the 57 might have liked it in practice. Ten of the 33 people in single rooms were private patients.

Reasons for preferring a room of their own were mainly a desire for peace and quiet, and various objections to other patients.

'If you're suffering from nervous trouble, you just want peace, and that's the last thing in the world you get while you're in hospital.' (In ward of 5–9 beds.)

'Well, I like quiet and that. I don't like gossip and those awful old wives' tales that frighten you. I think I would have been very much happier in a room of my own. I was very nervy, you know, and I felt I needed some real rest.'

'I'd prefer a room of my own if I had a bell, although people in a ward are friendly towards each other. It's a sort of community, but it's smelly, though I know it can't be avoided.'

'I like privacy. When I'm not feeling well I can't stand other people around. I don't like other people to witness my depression. I like to relax with my pain. I don't sleep very well and I read a great deal and to turn out my light at 9 p.m. and stop reading. . .'

'Even if it were a bit lonely at times I didn't mind that. I would have hated being in the ward at visiting hours and some of the people were so sick.'

Objections to noise were mentioned as a reason for their preference by a quarter of those who preferred a single room, by 29% of those who would have liked a ward which was smaller than the one they were in, and by 11% of those who were in and who preferred small wards of two to four beds. Another obvious reason given for their preference was their own personality—their shyness or gregariousness.

Summary and conclusions

What does all this add up to? One conclusion is that for most people the advantages of companionship with other patients outweigh the disadvantages. The last chapter showed that many patients had mixed feelings about each other, appreciating some aspects of their enforced proximity and intimacy and being made anxious by others. But only 8% of all patients wanted a room of their own. The majority said they preferred the size of ward they were in. There is, however, some indication that the anxiety, frustration and distress caused by other patients is less in small wards than in large ones.

Obviously patients' relationships with each other are only one of the considerations in planning ward size and layout. But, since an increasing proportion of patients are up and about for an appreciable part of their stay in hospital,[1] it becomes more practical to consider other arrangements. The best plan might be for all or most patients to have single rooms at night and when they are seriously ill, but to spend a large part of the day in common rooms with other patients. With such a scheme their reactions to a room of their own might be very different. If people can escape from or shut out the sight, the sound and the smell of the sick patient in the next bed, their ability to sympathize with and support each other is likely to be increased rather than diminished. But boredom, loneliness and apathy will beset people if they are isolated, and people confined to bed but not seriously ill need companionship. They are also likely to appreciate a change of scene, and a room of their own at night and a bed in a common room during the day might prove the best arrangement for them.

In the last three chapters the discussion about life in the ward has covered fears of death, embarrassment about bed-pans, irritation with strange habits, the friendliness of patients and the cheerfulness of nurses. This variety of topics is not entirely perverse or irrational, but reflects the diverse components of the day-to-day life in a hospital ward, where boredom is interspersed with drama and tragedy, loneliness is relieved by the companionship of strangers, the hopefulness of the convalescent contrasts with the hopelessness of the dying, the strangeness of a new environment is succeeded by the security of a known routine, and anxiety, hilarity and embarrassment intermingle with monotony.

When hospital buildings are old and ill-adapted to present-day circumstances, and hospital staff inadequate in number and overworked, many of the more distressing aspects of hospital life are inevitably accentuated. That patients adjust to this life as well as they do is a result of their own powers of adaptation, the kindness and sympathy of the nurses, and the friendship and support that patients give each other.

[1] Ministry of Health. *Report for the Year 1952, Part II*, p. 195, Jarrett, R. J., and Gazet, J. C., 'Aspects of Convalescence after Herniorrhaphy'.

PART THREE

The Problem of Communication

VI

THE DESIRE FOR INFORMATION

WHEN patients go into hospital they become part of a large and complex institution. They do this at a time when they are ill, so both their own condition and their environment are unfamiliar and in some ways unpleasant. It is a situation potentially full of anxiety. Pain, disability and even death are possibilities which confront them. How can anxiety be relieved and reality accepted?

Confidence in the hospital, the doctors and the nurses is obviously vital. But the ways in which confidence is built up clearly vary between doctors, between patients and between societies. When medicine was an art virtually unsupported by science the personality of the doctor and the patient's faith in him were all-important in creating confidence and trust. As science has been added to the art of comforting the foundations on which confidence is built have inevitably changed. Personalities are still often important, but many patients need information and explanations to support their trust in the medical profession. As Susser and Watson[1] put it, 'changes in education and culture led patients to expect scientific explanations from the doctor, and made them more aware of the nature both of his skills and of his limitations'. Some will accept treatment more readily when they understand its nature and purpose. For others, there is comfort to be found in surrender to what is seen as benevolent authority. For them the knowledge that they have been admitted to an institution geared to the care and treatment of the sick may be enough to enable them to relax and accept without question the procedures that their treatment entails.

Patients differ not only in the level of their interest in their illness and treatment, but also in their ability to understand and accept information. What is more, their needs for information are likely to

[1] Susser, M. W., and Watson, W., *Sociology in Medicine*, p. 178.

vary at different stages of their illness. How successful is the hospital in meeting this variety of needs?

Satisfaction with information

Altogether three-fifths of the patients interviewed reported some difficulty in getting information while they were in hospital. Twenty-one per cent said, in answer to a direct question, that they were unable to find out all they wanted to know about their condition, their treatment or their progress while they were in hospital.[1] A further 5% said they would have liked things explained to them in more detail,[2] another 3% said they were not able to find out about things as soon as they wanted to,[3] and an additional 13% made other comments which indicated that they were not entirely satisfied with the information they received.[4] Finally, a further 19% had had some difficulty in communication, since they had been unable to think of all the things they wanted to ask the doctors while they were there, and only thought of some things afterwards.[5]

Some of these patients may have been given explanations which they misunderstood, misinterpreted or even did not hear. For others, it may be that only after they left hospital did they realize there were things they had not fully understood or would have liked to have had explained more fully. Other patients again may not have been given certain information simply because no one had it—for example, they may have wanted a precise name for a condition which was undiagnosed. Hospital staff with enough time, opportunity, understanding and skill could realize, anticipate and overcome many of these sorts of difficulty. But some of the patients may have wanted not information and explanation but reassurance. If this could not be given, they needed help in adapting to changed circumstances.

Others may not have been given information because it was felt, for one reason or another, that it was better to withhold it from them. This raises a different problem—how far should the medical profession be prepared to make such decisions for their patients? One

[1] Question 53: 'While you were in hospital were you able to find out all you wanted to know about your condition, your treatment and your progress?'
[2] Question 54: 'Was there anything [else] you would have liked to have had explained in more detail?'
[3] Question 55: 'Were you able to find out about things as soon as you wanted to?'
[4] Comments arising at Questions 53–62 inclusive.
[5] Question 62: 'Did you find it easy to think of all the things you wanted to ask while the doctors were there or did you sometimes only think of things afterwards?'
N.B. Although all these questions were asked for each patient, they have been treated as mutually exclusive, in the order presented in the percentages quoted above.

relevant criterion for deciding this is whether or not patients accept and feel satisfied with the limited information or even misinformation they have been given.

Whatever the reasons, patients were more critical about the difficulty of obtaining information than of any other aspect of their hospital care. Whereas only 12% of the patients were not entirely satisfied with their medical treatment,[1] and 23% made some critical comment on the nursing, 61% described some failure of communication.[2] The implications of this failure depend on the kinds of information sought by patients and the importance they attach to it.

What do patients want to know?

The medical information patients want may be about their illness, its treatment or the prognosis. In practice these aspects are only rarely clearly differentiated, and most queries involve more than one. Thus, questions about the cause or nature of an illness are often either directly or implicitly—linked with queries about the likelihood of recurrence or probable development.

'I wanted to know why I kept having the abortions, but the doctors were too distant to talk to.'

'I'd like to have known just what was wrong with me, which kidney it was and if I'd be completely cured. Also I wanted to know if I could have any children. They just jump down your throat if you ask them.'

Other questions about the reason for treatment and the results of tests reveal doubts about the nature of their illnesses and the possible implications.

'I think I should have been told straight out why they had to do a total [hysterectomy]. There must have been some reason.'

'I had a heart specialist—he took an electrocardiograph of my heart. I asked him what was the matter. He said, "You'll be all right." I might just as well not have asked.'

Some patients described anxieties about particular illnesses or conditions they feared they or their babies might have.

'They don't really tell you enough. I saw on the baby's card something I didn't understand and I asked. They just said it meant that she was born

[1] Question 26: 'In general do you feel satisfied or dissatisfied with the medical treatment you received while you were in hospital?'
[2] The number of questions they were asked explains some of this variation, but not all of it. The proportions directly critical at the first question on the different subjects were 4% of their medical treatment, 3% of the nurses, and 21% of the information or lack of information.

the wrong way, but they didn't explain anything. And, of course, her little face was so damaged that the first few days her eyes were just slits —I thought she was a mongol. It wasn't until my husband said after about three days, "Is she a mongol?" that I managed to ask.'

'You don't like to ask too much and they're reluctant to tell you too much. I suppose if you say, "Doctor, have I got cancer?" they wouldn't tell you, would they? I didn't ask if it was cancerous. It was only a little lump—they removed the whole breast.'

Several people said they would have liked to have been told more about what was done and found at their operations.

'I would like to have been told after the operation what they had done like. All the staff were the type you couldn't speak to a lot really. When I did ask once they just said "Scrape". I don't know what that was except from hearing old wives' tales from other patients.'

'I'd like to have known all they had to do inside me. They didn't give any details. While I was at my brother's I saw the operation on telly and that told me more about it than they did. Now, if they had shown me a diagram and explained what they were going to do. I'm not all that daft. If he had said, "Now we are going to do this and that", I would have felt happier, but nobody said anything.' (Gall bladder removed.)

Anxieties about operations were often linked to their possible effect on sexual or reproductive capacity.

'Some patients said you could ask what the operation was, that you were allowed to ask. I asked sister then on the morning I was coming home. I would have liked to have known earlier. I was guessing—a living quiz programme. Sister said I could still have children—I'd like just one.' (Ovarian cyst.)

'I would like to know how the operation did go on—if they had taken away anything else at the operation unbeknown to me.' (A woman with appendicitis.)

Other queries were related to various effects on their lives in the future. 'How long I'd be off work'. 'How I could expect to be afterwards when I got out. How I'd be affected in time to come.' 'My work—how I would manage.' 'Would I get all right and would there be any repetitions.' 'What things like swimming I'd have to miss out on in the future.'

There were some direct questions about the results of tests and the purpose of treatment and other procedures.

'I'd like to have known actually what the blood was taken from me for. One and a half pints. They didn't explain. I'm a rare blood group. The consultant shook me by the hand and said, "We're very grateful for what you've done for us." They asked me in out-patients if I'd like to give a bit of blood. I said, "Certainly", but they didn't tell me anything.' (Had been in hospital to have some teeth extracted.)

'They would give you pills and if you asked what they were for you were told to take it and never mind. You were treated like a child, as if it was nothing to do with you if the medicine was changed. There was no reason given.'

'The type of food you can eat and what's best left alone. They tell you broadly and you keep on getting things that aren't on the diet sheet and you don't know whether you should eat them or not.'

A few patients complained that they were not told when things were going to be done to them.

'I didn't know I was going to have a blood transfusion. It gave me a bit of a shock. I felt better for it, though.'

'I would have liked to have been told *when* I was going down for the op., but they didn't. Nobody knew when we were going down. For six days this went on.'

The information which patients sought ranged over such varied topics as details of diet, significance of symptoms, purpose of pills, duration of disabilities, birth weights of babies, and capacity to copulate. The difficulties they describe are by no means confined to trivial or isolated incidents. What are the reasons for this failure in communication? One seems to be that patients hesitate to ask for the information they want.

The diffidence of patients

Many of the descriptions given by patients of their difficulties in communication revealed their own diffidence about questioning hospital staff.

'I didn't like the idea of asking. I thought I might be poking my nose into other people's affairs.'

'I left it to their generosity, you know, but they didn't tell me anything. They don't like you to ask them anything. You're there for treatment, you know. I would really have liked to get to know what was wrong with me and I guessed when they were putting blood into me it was for anaemia.'

Some seemed to feel that they could not expect explanations.

'They take us in to get better. You didn't ought to be too nosy. Those doctors in there—they're the ones to get us better.'

Others feared a rebuff.

'I didn't like to ask, perhaps it's just me. I felt they might think I was prying or being a bit nosy.'

'I learned indirectly the names of the tablets I was having. I gathered it was an understood thing that you didn't ask the doctor—they would take it amiss if you did. I wouldn't have had the audacity to ask sister in case of a snub. She might say, "It's none of your business to know what you're having." I don't know how sister and staff nurse would react if you asked them directly. It's a point I'm not sure about—whether you had a right to know.'

But in spite of this kind of diffidence, nearly half the patients felt they had asked for information more often than it was volunteered. In reply to the question: 'In general did you ask about things or did people tell you of their own accord?' 45% said they mainly asked, 40% that they were told, 7% that they neither asked nor were told, and 8% did not answer in these terms. A number of the comments of those who mainly asked show that they had found it was the only way to obtain any information.

'If you asked you always got to know. If you don't ask you don't get told.'

'You have to ask. They wouldn't tell you if you didn't ask.'

Some felt they had to explain or justify their action.

'I'm a cheeky devil, I used to ask. That's the only way to find out.'

'I had to ask the nurses on the sly. The doctors didn't tell me much.'

It seems that even those who mainly asked for information often had to overcome their diffidence first and even then some did not feel that asking had got them very far.

'You ask so much and then you're expected to guess the rest.'

'You have to ask. They will look at you and walk away without a word if you don't ask. At least they will just say "Good morning" and "Satisfactory". Even if you do ask, they don't tell you much.'

Dissatisfaction with the information they obtained was more often expressed by those who mainly asked than those who said people generally told them things of their own accord. Those who neither asked nor were told were the most dissatisfied. This is shown in Table 11.

The higher level of satisfaction among those who were mainly told things appears to be partly explained by a lower expectation and desire for information.

'I never asked about much. Mostly they'd come and tell you. They didn't give you the chance to ask them. They used more or less to tell you.'

'I never asked any questions, just left it to them to say. I wouldn't trouble them by asking questions.'

The Desire for Information

Some of these patients had been 'told things' indirectly by hearing discussions among the staff. 'I was mostly told. They weren't too bad. When the doctor examined me I heard what they said, so I didn't need to ask.' 'They hold a meeting round the bed. They told you as they talk among themselves.'

Occasionally the information they obtained in this way seemed to be concerned with the organization of the hospital rather than their own condition. 'With regard to the Institution, they tell you what is expected of you.' 'Anything to do with your condition they told you, and anything to do with the rules and regulations they told you quickly.'

There can be no doubt that many patients did feel diffident about asking questions, and although some overcame their diffidence on occasions, this reluctance to express their desire for information is a barrier to communication.

TABLE 11

SATISFACTION WITH INFORMATION AND HOW IT WAS OBTAINED

Attitude to information	How information obtained		
	Mainly asked	Mainly told	Neither asked nor told
	%	%	%
Not able to find out all they wanted to know	26	12	41
Other difficulty in communication ..	45	34	35
No difficulty in communication ..	29	54	24
Number of patients (= 100%) ..	323	291	49

Some reasons for patients' diffidence

Some reasons why patients might accept hospital procedures unquestioningly have already been suggested. These are their probable identification with the broad aims of the hospital, the strange and sometimes intimidating environment, and their own illness. When both their own condition and their environment are strange and new, and the general aims of the institution—to make them well again—are understood and accepted, people are more likely to adapt themselves to the institution than to try to change it. If they come across

79

attitudes or behaviour which they do not understand, they are probably more inclined to interpret them as necessary for the efficient functioning of the institution than to criticize them; if they sense that questions are not expected, they are apt to accept this and adjust to it.

There is also the problem of language. Patients may not know some of the terms which doctors use, and they may misinterpret others. They may feel inhibited about expressing their problems if they can only do so readily in terms which doctors do not use. These difficulties may be intensified when the hospital staff come from other countries. One patient said: 'The houseman when I went in examined me and told me what was wrong in Arabic.' Then, too, patients may not understand or may have misconceptions about physiological or anatomical details while doctors may assume that these are understood. And, when so many patients are diffident about asking doctors straightforward questions, they are likely to be reluctant to expose their ignorance.

Another contributory cause is the awe with which some patients regard the doctors.

'I didn't like to ask. You can't get through to them, you know—they seem a bit above you.'

'You're a bit nervous of these big doctors and specialists.'

'Mr. ——'s a bit awe-inspiring. You forget what you want to ask.'

Social distance between doctors and patients contributes to this feeling. Table 12 shows that patients in the professional class were more likely to ask questions, while those in the unskilled manual group more often waited to be told.[1]

A similar difference was observed by Freidson[2] in a survey of Medical Group subscribers in New York: 'High social class was associated with a greater degree of sensitivity to social stimuli in the doctor-patient relationship, and with a critical and manipulative approach to medical care. In contrast, the lower classes were less sensitive about their status as patients and were rather more passive and uncritical in their approach to medical care.'

The tendency to regard doctors as unapproachable may be decreasing. Younger people were more prepared to ask questions than older people (see Table 13), but this difference could be explained by patients becoming more passive and feeling they are more likely to be told unwelcome facts as they get older.

There is no doubt that the prestige of doctors in the community is

[1] For a description of the classification of social class see Appendix 6.
[2] Freidson, E., *Patients' Views of Medical Practice*, pp. 210–11.

The Desire for Information

TABLE 12

SOCIAL CLASS VARIATIONS
IN HOW PATIENTS OBTAINED INFORMATION

How information obtained	Social class				
	Professional	Other non-manual*	Skilled manual	Partly skilled	Unskilled
	%	%	%	%	%
Mainly asked	65	53	49	45	40
Mainly told ..	31	41	44	49	50
Neither asked nor told ..	4	6	7	6	10
Number of patients (= 100%) ..	23	180	232	130	50

* This includes Intermediate Class II and non-manual workers included in the Registrar-General's Class III. If these were shown separately the trend would not be so clear-cut. The proportion who mainly asked was 47% in Class II and 63% in Class III non-manual.

TABLE 13

VARIATIONS WITH AGE
IN HOW PATIENTS OBTAINED INFORMATION

How information obtained	Patient's age*		
	Under 45	45–64	65 or more
	%	%	%
Mainly asked	60	41	35
Mainly told	33	53	53
Neither asked nor told	7	6	12
Number of patients (= 100%) ..	303	236	122

* If smaller age groups are taken, the proportion who 'mainly asked' is 59%, 62%, 40%, 43%, and 35% for the groups 21–34, 35–44, 45–54, 55–64, and 65 and over, respectively.

81

very high,[1] and there may be some people who become inarticulate when confronted by a white coat or a stethoscope. One or two described instances of 'doctor-fright'.

'It seems as if you dry up when the doctor comes. He says "How are you?" and you say "all right" even if you feel bleeding awful.'

'I was strung up when the doctors were there, and forgot things.'

'You get hot and bothered when they're there and think afterwards "I wish I'd asked them that." '

On the other hand, familiarity with the television hospital ward can lead to critical comparisons.

'None of the doctors explained things—not like Emergency Ward 10.'

A feeling of respect towards the medical profession, though it can obviously contribute to a sense of security, can sometimes become a barrier to adequate communication. Deference and diffidence may conceal a desire for explanation or information, so that hospital staff are unaware of it.

Passivity and acceptance

How many patients are passive accepters? Although this question implies an immense oversimplification of a complex problem, it is probably worth posing in this form, since conceptions about the proportion of such patients can influence the attitudes and ideas of hospital staff about the importance of explanations.

In an attempt to throw some light on this problem patients were asked: 'When you are ill, do you like to know as much as possible about what is wrong with you—or how do you feel?'[2] Three-quarters of the patients said they liked to know as much as possible, while most of the others gave replies which indicated that they did not want to know too much. Some of the latter answered the question generally —'I don't like to think about it', 'The more you know the more it worries you', 'The less I know the better', 'Just a little bit! I don't like to know too much'. Others qualified their responses by such phrases as 'Not if I had anything really serious', 'If I had only six months to live I wouldn't want to know', 'Well, if it was anything such as something I wasn't going to get over I'd rather stay in the dark. I wouldn't like to be told if I had cancer. I don't think I could live with that.'

[1] Hall, J., and Jones, D. C., 'Social Grading of Occupations', and Young, M., and Willmott, P., 'Social Grading by Manual Workers'.
[2] Question 60; This question could no doubt have been better put. It is almost a leading question, possibly encouraging people to say that they like to know as much as possible, rather than explain how they feel.

The Desire for Information

A further question divided those who wanted to know as much as possible into those who said they were mainly interested in how it affected them, two-fifths of the total sample, and those who wanted to know the details as well, one-third of those interviewed.[1]

The extent to which people were satisfied with the information they received was clearly related to how much they wanted to know. Explicit expression of dissatisfaction was twice as common among those who wanted to know as much as possible as among other patients, but the others were almost as likely to express indirect criticism. This can be seen from Table 14.

TABLE 14

ATTITUDES TO INFORMATION AND DESIRE FOR INFORMATION

Attitude to information	How much wanted to know		
	As much as possible		Not as much as possible
	including details	but mainly how it affects me	
	%	%	%
Not able to find out all they wanted to know	27	23	11
Other difficulty in communication	46	39	37
No difficulty in communication	27	38	52
Number of patients (= 100%)	236	297	142

Even so, nearly half of the patients who did not want to know as much as possible described some way in which they had found it difficult to get what information they did want, and a third of them felt that they had asked for information more often than the staff had given it spontaneously.

The proportion of patients who were consistently passive—who did not want to know too much, did not ask for information, and described no difficulty in communication—was 10%. 'I put myself in their hands', and 'They never said anything. I trusted in them; they'd done it before to lots of people', were comments made by two people in this group.

[1] Question 61: 'Are you mainly interested in how it is going to affect you or do you like to know the actual mechanical details as well?' Organic or physiological details would have been a more appropriate wording, but mechanical was found to be more readily understood.

A larger group of patients, the 33% who said they wanted to know as much as possible, including the details, made such remarks as:

'I don't like to think there's something going on and I don't know.'

'I feel better knowing. You always imagine things are worse than they are.'

'I hate being kept in the dark. I like to know every mortal thing about it.

'I hate being treated like a fool.'

'If I had an incurable disease I'd like to be told.'

Several of the 42% who wanted to know as much as possible, but were mainly interested in how it affected them, also put the view that 'it's better to know than to surmise'. Other comments were:

'I'm not interested in the details of operations, but I like to know what it involves and what to expect.'

'When I'm confronted with something that I don't understand, I like to know as much about it as possible—the danger of complications, the possibility of survival—what it's all leading up to—an overall prospect; I don't want the job filleted.'

So, although many patients felt hesitant about questioning hospital staff about their illness or treatment, this was not usually because of indifference or desire to be left in ignorance; and the passive or even 'ostrich-like' reaction of a small group of patients may itself be partly promoted and encouraged by the attitude of some hospital staff. It is possible that if some of these patients were encouraged to take a more constructive interest in their treatment and condition they would be able to adjust more readily to the realities of their condition and its possible handicaps. Coser[1] has noted that the passive patient facilitates treatment, but resists recovery; the active patient may interfere with treatment, but is better equipped to recover.

Appreciation of information

Not all patients were either passive accepters or dissatisfied with the information they obtained. A quarter of all those interviewed said that they both liked to know as much as possible about their illness and had no difficulty in obtaining the information they wanted. Illustrations of their appreciation are given below:

'What I liked about the specialist was that he told you exactly what was happening, what was causing it and what they were going to do about it.'

'I was very fortunate. Dr. —— treats his patients as intelligent people. A lot of doctors don't believe in it.'

[1] Coser, R., 'A Home Away from Home'.

'When the doctor came round to see you, you could always ask, and he told me. If they were going to do anything they told you what it would be like and why they were doing it—that's what I liked. There was a hard covering over my heart restricting the muscles. I asked him how he'd done the operation and he told me they'd peeled the hard covering off, like skinning an old rabbit. What more could a man say to me explaining?'

Table 15, which shows the association between patients' satisfaction with their treatment and with the information they received, suggests that explanations help patients to accept the need for medical treatment.

TABLE 15

DISSATISFACTION WITH MEDICAL TREATMENT
AND SATISFACTION WITH INFORMATION

Attitude to medical treatment	Attitude to information		
	Not able to find out all they wanted to know	Other difficulty in communication	No difficulty in communication
	%	%	%
Satisfied	74	89	95
Dissatisfied ..	12	3	—
Uncertain, or qualified	14	8	5
Number of patients (= 100%)	149	287	283

Dissatisfaction was expressed much more frequently by the patients who said they were unable to find out all that they wanted to know than by those who had no complaints on that score. Putting this another way round, two-thirds of those who were dissatisfied with their medical treatment said they were unable to find out all they wanted to know, compared with a fifth of those who said they were entirely satisfied.

This emphasizes the importance of personal relationships in determining patients' attitudes towards medical treatment. More pragmatically, it shows the importance of giving patients adequate explanations if doctors are to maintain or acquire a good clinical reputation amongst their patients.

The Problem of Communication

Summary and conclusions

Over half the patients described some difficulty in getting information while they were in hospital. While it can be argued that some patients may have forgotten, not accepted or misunderstood what they were told, and others were really seeking reassurance or even misinformation, there is evidence of a serious failure of communication between some patients and hospital staff. This failure is both obscured and accentuated by patients' acceptance of authoritarian views and practices, their low level of expectation, and their diffidence about questioning hospital staff. Authoritarian attitudes tend to become self-perpetuating once accepted, and it may take unusually persistent patients or particularly perceptive doctors to change them. If people do not ask for explanations, it is tempting to assume that they do not want them.

Staff and patients need to interpret their respective roles in the same way if there is to be adequate communication between them. If the doctor assumes that his role is to diagnose and treat the patient's condition and to give any explanation about this that the patient asks for, this will work efficiently only if the patient clearly understands that he must ask for any explanations he wants. The illustrations have shown that many patients do not interpret their role in this way, but hope that doctors or nurses will explain things of their own accord.

When patients are diffident about asking for the information they want, then it is crucial that the hospital staff themselves should recognize patients' needs. Clearly this task calls for understanding, skill, patience, experience and time. The role of medical and nursing staff in providing patients with information are discussed in the next chapters. The comments of the patients interviewed suggest that the task is even more difficult than hospital staff often appreciate, and that too little attention is paid to it, both in the general organization of hospital routine and in the medical curricula.

VII

DOCTORS AS A SOURCE OF INFORMATION

So far this discussion of communication between patients and staff has been concerned mainly with patients' attitudes—with their desire for information, and their diffidence about questioning hospital staff. This chapter and the next describe their sources of information and the ways in which the relationships between patients and staff influence the ease with which they communicate.

Forty-six per cent of the patients said their main source of information had been a doctor; for 28% it was the sister, for 11% a nurse, and for 2% the other patients. Seven per cent said they had not received any information from anyone and were critical about this, and 4% maintained they had not needed any information. Two per cent mentioned various other sources including physiotherapists, ward orderlies, students, the matron and 'the chart at the bottom of the bed'.[1]

The medical staff were thus the most frequent source of information, and a further 32% of the patients, though they did not describe the doctors as their main source of information, said, in answer to a later question,[2] that they had found some doctors helpful in this way. Twenty-one per cent had not found any doctors helpful.

It was not possible to ascertain the rank of doctor mentioned by a quarter of those who said their main source of information was a doctor, but among those for whom it could be traced 54% were consultants, 27% house officers, 12% registrars and 7% clinical assistants.

Some comments from patients with these different sources of information are given below, beginning with those who regarded the

---

[1] Question 56: 'Who did you find out most about your condition, your treatment and your progress from—while you were in hospital?'

[2] Question 56 (cont.) IF DOCTOR NOT MENTIONED: 'What about the doctors—which of them was most helpful in this way?'

doctors as their main source of information. They illustrate the type of relationship that existed in these situations, and how the patients felt about it.

'You'd just to ask him and he'd tell you in words of three letters. He was very good explaining about sexual intercourse after the operation [for prolapse] without being embarrassing.' (House officer most helpful.)

'He was informative, he would tell you things quite frankly.' (Consultant most helpful.)

'She breezes in and out. If you can nail her down she talks.' (Clinical assistant most helpful.)

Comments from patients who found some doctors helpful, but did not regard them as their main source of information included:

'The professor told me most of what I wanted to know—that the lump was quite all right. But I also wanted to know what had been done and I asked the sister and she told me exactly. I should say she told me most for the simple reason it was her I asked the most.'

'I respect doctors but I don't sort of hold conversations with them.' (Nurse main source—house officer most helpful of doctors.)

And from those who did not find any doctors helpful:

'You didn't have much to do with them. They give you a nod and stand chatting to sister at the foot of the bed. They are rather like gods in hospital. I think if you did ask they would tell you anything.' (Sister main source.)

'Oh no, they don't tell you anything—just that you've got to have it off. [Growth in breast.] And when he came in to see us after he just said, "Well it's gone now." I didn't ask the surgeon what kind of growth it was.' (Other patients main source.)

'The doctors came round one Sunday morning. Five yards away they'd forgotten about you. Same as in prison—you're just a number. They walk away and forget about you.' (No one helpful.)

Once again the diffidence of patients is illustrated, but these comments also show how the circumstances in which doctors and patients meet in hospital can influence communications.

Ward rounds

A number of patients described the ward rounds in terms which illustrate the difficulties of talking to the doctors then.

'The consultant came round with an assistant and students, explaining cases. The doctor looked at me, said nothing and asked the students to examine me and find out what was the matter. They seemed to find out, but they didn't tell me.'

'They examine you and wander off in the distance without telling you how you are getting on.'

'I'd like to have known what caused me to be like that. But it was my fault, dear, I was to blame. I didn't ask. The surgeon saw me twice. When they come round the head's there and the other doctors are listening, learning from the head doctor. You feel a bit embarrassed. Some doctors are a bit sarcastic.'

Some comments suggest that doctors, concentrating on teaching or immersed in intellectual or technical problems of diagnosis or treatment, may behave in a way which appears arrogant to patients.

'There's a lot of talk going on and very little said to the patient to put his mind at rest. The doctor and sister are talking at the bed. I think they should either go away and have the discussion elsewhere, or the patient should be brought into the discussion. If you were to ask, I had the feeling you'd be told to mind your own business.'

'The surgeon came round with a lot of students and you could hear what they were saying. It was a bit rough on some others in the ward; they were more or less made an object of. The surgeon demonstrates and the students have to diagnose. In most cases this is very painful for the patient. They stood at the bed and discussed you quite openly. They found out what was wrong with themselves in medical terms; they didn't get a lot of facts. The patient speaks and the only answer is: "You're doing very well. We'll have you out in no time." '

'When they are talking in technical terms across your body you would like to know what is being said. These long Latin names—one wonders what they mean.'

Several patients described their embarrassment and confusion when confronted by a group of doctors on a ward round.

'I had a sort of a blank, you know, especially when you have five or six round you and when they're young, too, and you're stripped. You sort of dry up and don't know whether to say it or not, when there's two or three, in case they think you're soppy.'

'The position is that when the doctors come round and you're like that —prone, and so you have six bodies towering over you. It's rather unfavourable, so some things escape you.'

Such circumstances are hardly conducive to discussion, and obviously increase the patients' reluctance to ask the doctors questions. An unhurried atmosphere of intimacy and privacy is necessary to overcome the diffidence and embarrassment which so many patients feel in talking to doctors. Some patients had come across arrangements which were more helpful.

'You're an entity and you're known by name and you call the doctors "Doc". It's very easy to get to them, none of these formalities. You can always have an interview and can have a man-to-man talk with them. They told you step by step what was wrong and what they were going to do.'

'They said immediately what had to be done and the surgeon came round more or less as soon as you were awake and told you what had been done.'

But these experiences were comparatively rare; most patients described either formal ward rounds or hurried routine visits. The former seem particularly likely to intimidate patients and to create an impression of the omnipotence and inaccessibility of the doctor.

The attitudes of doctors

Several patients did not find the attitudes of the doctors helpful when they were asked questions.

'They say, in the pamphlet they give you, you can always ask the doctor questions, but they made me feel I was a hypochondriac when I asked simple questions.'

'I had a feeling they just thought you were a nuisance if you asked questions. I did ask to see the afterbirth, but Dr. —— said, "Oh, you don't want to see that", and that was that. It's always an education to see things like that, and you know people take the trouble to find out about it now and they know much more about it. I read all I could about it.'

It is difficult for patients to overcome their diffidence when the doctors are not encouraging, and many patients found them unapproachable.

'The specialists don't seem to have mastered the art of personal relationships. They remain aloft—don't want to talk too much. When you find him jumping over your questions it makes you lose confidence.'

'One of the doctors was most abrupt. You don't like to ask them.'

Pratt, Seligmann and Reader[1] showed that doctors tend to underestimate the knowledge of their patients, and that physicians who seriously underestimated this knowledge were less likely to discuss the illness at any length than others. A number of patients we interviewed felt the staff regarded them as uneducated, unintelligent or unable to understand explanations.

[1] Pratt, L., Seligmann, A., and Reader, G., 'Physicians' Views on the Level of Medical Information among Patients'.

'Well, I was worried whether having this stuff in my water would affect the baby, but the sister just said, "You're worrying yourself unduly. You should leave these things to us." But I don't think she thought I could understand. I think she thought I wasn't educated enough.'

'They leave you in the dark too much. If only they treated you as if you could understand something. The doctors especially were very superior; they didn't tell you anything.'

'The attitude of the medical profession that's still prevalent is: "You're not intelligent enough to know what you're taking." '

Some described how they felt they had been fobbed off with trite statements.

'They don't tell you anything—only that you're doing all right—that sort of thing.'

And there were other forms of evasion.

'I thought of all sorts of things, but they don't like you to ask. When you do ask them anything they say: "We'll come to that in a minute"—but that minute never comes. They ask *you* the questions.'

'You get side-tracked. They don't answer direct.'

Thus it seems to patients that some doctors discourage them from asking questions. They use the patients' feelings of deference and respect to evade discussion. They appear to do this partly because they do not appreciate their patients' need for explanations, partly because they underestimate their ability to understand explanations, and also because they wish to protect themselves from personal involvement with their patients' problems.

The impersonality of the doctor

When a patient goes into hospital he is normally under a consultant, who is clinically responsible for him. It is indeed quite customary in hospital to describe a patient as 'belonging to' a consultant. The general practitioner will often refer a patient to a particular consultant and the consultant's name is frequently put on a card by the patient's bed. Hospital staffing is hierarchical, with consultants and senior hospital medical officers at the top, followed by senior registrars, registrars, senior house officers and house officers. These various grades are not distinguished by titles nor by dress, so that the patient may be unaware of the structure of the organization and of the doctors' relative positions. Although he is formally under a consultant, it is possible that he may never see him personally and much of the examination and day-to-day care of routine cases will be carried out by more junior staff. To what extent does this arrangement give patients a sense of identification and personal relationship with the doctors with whom they come into contact?

Most of the patients, 70%, were prepared to identify a person they felt was their particular hospital doctor.[1] The rank of the doctor they selected varied widely, and not all of them were able to tell us who 'their particular doctor' was. Altogether 29% mentioned a consultant or senior hospital medical officer, 13% a houseman, 6% a registrar and 5% a clinical assistant. Five per cent of them mentioned a name which we were unable to trace and 12% were unable to tell us the name or rank.[2]

Factors which appeared important in creating a feeling of identification were the frequency with which patients saw the doctor, the ease with which they felt they could discuss things with him, the prestige or authority of the doctor, and previous contact with him before they were admitted to hospital. Some patients stressed other aspects of their relationship with 'their hospital doctor'.

'A little black doctor. He had a lovely smile. It made you feel better just to see him. He seemed to have more patience. He was bright and cheerful. Others would come and look that stern you expected the worst.'

'Dr. ——. He was most helpful. He filled in sheets and sheets of paper about me, like you're doing now, and asking questions.'

'Mr. ——, a very nice gentleman. He never said a lot, but you could see he was interested in the people he attended.'

'Dr. ——. He was young and nice-looking. He gave confidence to the youngsters. We used to watch them playing tennis.'

The different attributes they mentioned here suggest a possible conflict of loyalties or identification. Patients may see the house officer most frequently, but recognize that it is the consultant who is ultimately responsible for taking decisions. It is the consultant whom

---

[1] Question 64: 'Did you feel there was one doctor who was your particular hospital doctor? Who was that?'

[2] In the majority of instances the rank has been taken from the names the patient gave us and from lists of hospital staff which were obtained from the secretaries of the Hospital Management Committees concerned, but in a number of cases, 12%, the patient's own assessment of rank has been used. In the 91 instances when the patients quoted both a name and rank for the same doctor and this could be checked against the hospital list it was found that 79% were correct, but it is, of course, possible that some of the patients correctly related a name and rank, but attached them both to the wrong person. It was registrars who caused the most confusion; just over half of them were ascribed to the wrong rank and they were more likely to be 'demoted' to housemen than 'promoted' to consultants.

they are most likely to have seen previously,[1] but if they see him only on formal ward rounds they may find it easier to talk to the houseman.

Many of those who did not feel there was a doctor who was their particular one remarked on the number they had seen.

'There were so many understudies.'

'You haven't got one. Any Tom, Dick or Harry—I don't know where they all come from.'

'We had so many come through. You had one darkie and one white one day, and someone with glasses and an Oxford accent the next.'

Others were not prepared to identify one particular doctor, because they felt that all of them had been helpful.

'Each one was as nice as the other. They were all out to do what they could for you.'

'They all seemed interested. They all treated you like you were their patient.'

Those who felt they had a particular hospital doctor were no more likely to say they had been able to find out all they wanted to know than those who did not have that feeling, although the two groups did differ in the extent to which they had found doctors helpful as a source of information, as can be seen in Table 16.

Nearly a fifth of those saying they had a particular hospital doctor had reported earlier in the interview that none of the doctors had been helpful about giving them information. What seems most likely is that, because these patients saw a particular doctor regularly or frequently, or knew that he was the senior doctor in charge of the patients in his ward, they felt that they had a particular hospital doctor, but their relationship was not as intimate or personal as this phrase might seem to imply. Over a tenth of the people who said they had such a doctor had never known his name, and rather more had known it, but had forgotten it by the time they were interviewed. They may have identified a doctor merely because they felt this was the expected answer to our question, but also they may have felt a need for such a person. Identification of 'my doctor' can perhaps give some sense of security and of personal involvement, even though he only nods from the foot of the bed.

[1] Of those who had previously attended the out-patient department for the condition for which they were admitted, 71% had seen a doctor there whom they met subsequently in hospital, and the great majority of these, 48% in all, had seen the consultant compared with 8% a houseman, 6% a registrar and 3% a clinical assistant. In 17% of the cases the rank could not be ascertained, and 13% mentioned more than one doctor.

TABLE 16

IDENTIFICATION WITH A PARTICULAR HOSPITAL DOCTOR
AND DOCTORS AS A SOURCE OF INFORMATION

Doctors as source of information	*Felt had particular hospital doctor*	*Did not feel had particular hospital doctor*
	%	%
Doctors main source ..	50	39
Doctors helpful, but not main source	33	33
No doctors helpful	17	28
Number of patients (= 100%)	486	209

Another 'symptom' of the lack of personal relationship is that doctors only rarely introduce themselves to the patients, who generally find out their names by other, and sometimes unreliable, means. All the patients were asked this question: 'In general did the doctors tell you their names when you first saw them or how did you find them out?' Their replies are shown in Table 17.

The most common sources of this information were other patients and nurses. The doctors had introduced themselves to only 7% of the

TABLE 17
FINDING OUT DOCTORS' NAMES

Method	%
Never found them out	15
From other patients	25
From nurses	24
Had known doctor previously ..	14
From general practitioner ..	9
Name was on appointment card	8
Name was on chart over bed ..	7
Doctors introduced themselves..	7
Patient asked doctor	1
Other sources	12
Number of patients (= 100%) ..	709

22% of patients gave more than one answer.

patients and only 1% of the patients had asked the doctors directly. Some comments about this are given below.

'Through talk—through the other patients. You had a card over your bed with the specialist's name on it, but not his understudies' names. The card is a marvellous system—you feel you belong.'

'They didn't tell me their names and I didn't find them out. I asked the other patients and they didn't know, so it didn't worry me after that.'

'You find them out off the male sister. He used to say: "Dr. —— will be round today." I always thought it would be better if they said: "I'm Dr. ——", and then you'd know. But they don't do that. You can go into hospital and not know their names at all.'

It might be argued that doctors do not introduce themselves to patients either because patients already know who they are or because it is not necessary for them to know. The first argument is demonstrably false in many instances, and the second is questionable. If you know a person's name this helps to identify the person and to create a more personal relationship.[1] Normally middle-class people[2] are introduced, or introduce themselves, to people with whom they have a relationship which is at all personal. That hospital doctors largely ignore this convention in their dealings with patients suggests that they do not regard the relationship as a particularly personal one. It may be, too, that they feel there are advantages in an anonymous, professional relationship. Some conflict between the patient's desire for a personal relationship and the doctor's need to maintain a professional one is inevitable on occasions.[3] Our evidence suggests, though, that some hospital doctors could perform their professional role rather more effectively if they had a more personal relationship with their patients.

Particular problems of surgical patients

Further support for this last suggestion comes from the group of surgical patients in our sample. They were asked whether they had seen the surgeon and the anaesthetist before and after their operations. Their answers are shown in Table 18. Their statements may not

[1] Among those who said they never found out the doctors' names a comparatively low proportion, half, said they felt they had a particular hospital doctor, compared with three-quarters of those who had found out their names, and among those who felt they had a particular hospital doctor, the proportion saying that the doctors had been helpful in providing information was 85% among those who knew and remembered his name and 74% among those who felt they had one but did not know his name.

[2] Which most doctors are by upbringing as well as profession.

[3] For a discussion of this see Freidson, E., op. cit., chapter on 'Dilemmas in the Doctor-Patient Relationship'.

always be accurate, but what the patients thought happened is obviously of some importance in itself.

TABLE 18

CONTACT WITH THE SURGEON AND ANAESTHETIST
BEFORE AND AFTER OPERATION
(Surgical patients only)

	Proportion seeing:	
	Surgeon	*Anaesthetist*
	%	%
Before operation only	5	24
After operation only	19	4
Both before and after	60	13
Not at all	10	53
Did not know	6	6
Number of patients (= 100%) ..	354	

They were much more likely to have seen the surgeon than the anaesthetist, but a third went to the operating theatre without apparently having seen or identified the person who was to perform the operation. A number of those who had seen him made comments which showed that they had appreciated the personal contact and the opportunity to ask him questions. 'I saw the surgeon the night before and the morning after the operation. That was very, very good. I felt I knew him before I went down to the theatre.' 'Eleven o'clock at night I saw him. Lovely chat we had.' 'He came to me the night before the operation and we had a jolly good chat—that was the Indian doctor—the R.S.O. As far as I knew he was at the operation'. This last remark suggests that patients may sometimes have assumed which doctor did the operation on rather slender evidence. Other comments of those who had seen the surgeon indicate that they had a rather distant relationship with him. 'I saw them afterwards just. Two or three doctors came with the nurse and almoner. I didn't see them close. They said, "You've been lucky—you'll be all right." ' 'He just passed the bed and said, "Nasty appendix", that's all.'

A number of people who had not found out who operated on them rather resented this. 'I don't know who's done the job. I asked when I went for a check-up and saw the house surgeon. I only wanted to know so as to thank him. I asked the house surgeon who did it and he said, "Oh, one of the doctors in the hospital." Well, that was the brush-off. You feel you're treading on their toes and you don't want to irritate them.' 'They don't tell you really. When I went to the hospital before, at out-patients, I saw Professor ——, but he has a lot of doctors working under him and there was one came and inspected my legs and marked them up, but I don't know whether he was the one who did the operation. I think it would be better if they did tell you who was doing the operation. It would make you feel better, but they don't really tell you anything'.[1]

Those who had seen the surgeon were, not surprisingly, less likely to complain that they were not able to find out all they wanted to know (see Table 19).

TABLE 19

SATISFACTION WITH INFORMATION
AND CONTACT WITH SURGEON
(Surgical patients only)

	Surgeon seen:			
Satisfaction with information	*Before and after operation*	*Before or after not both*	*Neither*	*Did not know*
	%	%	%	%
Not able to find out all they wanted to know	13	19	28	31
Other difficulty in communication	43	38	36	43
No difficulty in communication	44	43	36	26
Number of patients (= 100%)	211	84	36	23

But even though two-thirds of patients had seen the surgeon before their operation, few of them had discussed their fears and anxieties with him. Altogether 16% said they had been very anxious, a third a little anxious, while half said they were not at all anxious before their operation. Those who expressed any anxiety were asked if they had discussed their worries with anyone either in hospital or before they went in. Over half, 57%, said they had not talked to anyone about it. 'I wouldn't let anyone see it' was a typical comment. Other patients

[1] The Parliamentary Secretary to the Ministry of Health, Mr. Bernard Braine, maintained in answer to a question in the House of Commons that 'there should be no difficulty in the patient finding out who performed the operation'.

were the most frequent confidants of those who had discussed their anxieties with anyone. 'I felt a little anxious, as I'd never had anything like that before. I had a talk to a chap who'd had it. He said, "Don't worry at all, mate." I felt better.' Sixteen per cent of those who felt at all anxious had talked to other patients about this, 13% had discussed their fears with friends or relatives, 8% with nurses or sister, 6% with hospital doctors and 2% with their general practitioner.

The comments of those who said they had not been at all anxious fall into three broad groups. For some the lack of anxiety seems connected with their own personality; for others with relief that something was to be done about their condition, and, for others again, with their relationship with hospital medical staff. Illustrations from this last group, which is the one relevant to this discussion, are:

'I just had confidence in them. I wasn't at all worried about it. They put you at ease so quickly. They're not at all straitlaced up there.'

'Mr. — gave me that confidence that everything was going to be all right. He was going to do the worrying for me. He sort of knew me and I knew him before the operation from visits to the ward. He talked about my family. It's a great thing. You feel you're not cut off. He never made you feel as though he was in a hurry. It was as though he was completely at leisure, although I knew he could ill afford the few minutes he spent with me.'

One occasion on which such anxieties might be discussed and possible questions answered is when patients sign the form consenting to the operation. An example of such a form is given below:

'I agree to the operation advised including, if necessary, the administration of an anaesthetic, and any further operation which you may consider necessary.

'I understand that no assurance has been given that the operation will be performed by any one particular surgeon.'

Signing such a form can be quite a terrifying thing for some people. 'I thought I was signing my death warrant.' One or two patients explained the reason for the form in terms which indicated that it had made them think of the possibility of dying. 'Your people won't think they've killed you without permission.' 'You excuse them if you die— it puts them in the clear.' Others appeared to accept it in a more matter-of-fact way. 'I just thought "I'm in now. I can't walk out". It didn't bother me. I'd made up my mind.'

Thirty-nine per cent of the patients had been given this form to sign by the sister, 29% by a nurse, 10% by a doctor, 5% by someone else, such as a receptionist, almoner or secretary, and the remaining 17% could not remember who gave it to them or could not recall signing.

Doctors as a Source of Information

The occasion was sometimes used for explanations about what was to be done and the reason for it.

'The sister gave it to me. She was good. She said, "We aren't going to take anything away and even if we do find anything we won't do anything until we have your further consent. It's just for the anaesthetic." I was impressed. It wasn't just thrust at you; it was really talked over.'

'The sister—she was very nice. She made sure I read it first.'

But for other patients it was part of a formal routine with little or no opportunity for discussion. 'As I was going in they told me to sign some papers. I was in such a state, so I don't know what I signed.' 'The sister just threw the card on to the bed and said "Put your name to that", and when I had she grabbed the form and was off.' 'A clerk gave it to me—I felt a little off-put by that.' And one patient who had been given the form by a nurse doing her training maintained, 'They always give it to you after your injection. You don't care then.'

The needs of surgical patients for information are probably more clearly defined than those of other patients, since much of the information they seek is related to the actual operation—its purpose, what was found, what was done, and the probable effect. Such an organized procedure as an operation[1] also provides some definite opportunities for explanation. This should make it easier in surgical than in medical wards to lay down an appropriate procedure which would ensure that all surgical patients other than emergencies were given at any rate basic information about their operation. Ideally all patients would be seen beforehand by the surgeon, who would explain the purpose of the operation. This would not only help to improve communications, but would increase clinical efficiency. The Medical Defence Union and the Royal College of Nursing recommended such a procedure in order to reduce the risk of a surgeon performing an operation on the wrong patient, side, limb or digit.[2] If the surgeon also gave the patient the consent form to sign when he was explaining the nature and purpose of the operation, this could provide a helpful basis for their discussion, whereas at the moment it is often just a legal formality. Afterwards, as one patient put it, 'You'd think the doctor that did the operation would come and have a talk to you.'

Summary

Although doctors are the most important source of information for patients, there are several aspects of the relationship between patients and hospital medical staff which make communication

---

[1] Seventy-two per cent of the surgical patients in the sample were admitted from the waiting list.

[2] *Joint Memorandum.*

between them difficult. The circumstances under which they meet in hospital are likely to increase patients' difficulties, because they emphasize the prestige and power of the doctors. Doctors tend to underestimate both patients' desire for information and their ability to understand explanations. They often seem to discourage patients from asking questions and they sometimes use the patients' feelings of respect and deference to evade discussion. The present arrangements do not encourage a personal relationship between patients and hospital doctors. If communications are to be improved, some doctors need to be more approachable people, less like inaccessible gods.

VIII

OTHER SOURCES OF INFORMATION

ALTHOUGH doctors were the most common source of information, less than half the patients altogether said they got most of their information from doctors. The other people who told them about their illness, treatment or progress are discussed in this chapter, starting with the sister.

The sister

The ward sister is a key person in the hospital communication network, the main link between medical and nursing staff, between senior administrative staff and nurses, and often between doctors and patients.

Just over a quarter of the patients said that the sister had been their main source of information. All the patients were asked whether she had given them a lot, a little or no information about their illness, treatment and progress.[1] Sixteen per cent said a lot, 40% a little and 44% none. Among those who said the sister was their main source of information, two-fifths said she gave them a lot of information and three-fifths a little.

Patients were asked what sort of things the sister told them about, and some examples are given below. First, from those who said she gave them a lot of information.

'She told me about what actually happened, that they had removed 13 gallstones but not the appendix.'

'On the morning I went in the sister explained to me what the doctor was going to do. And then on the morning after the operation she came and said that they'd had to do a lot more, but try not to worry and it would be all right.'

[1] Question 57: 'What about the sister—did she give you a lot of information, a little information or no information about your illness, treatment and progress? What sort of things did she tell you about?'

101

The Problem of Communication

For some of these patients the sister appeared to act as an interpreter of the doctor to the patient; she was more approachable or more able to express things in terms the patients could understand.

'She talks to the doctors and she could put it in a better way. She'd tell you anything you wanted to know. I wanted to know if I'd have another operation for that kidney and why I had blue dye in my arm. The sister was so interested in your personal affairs that I told her I had a lot of stairs to my flat, that I had to go down for every drop of water and that. She said she'd talk to the surgeon for me to see if I could get a ground-floor flat.'

Illustrations from patients who said the sister gave them a little information suggest that the information was sometimes fairly limited in scope but straightforward.

'When I was going to have the op., when I could have a bath, when I was going to have my stitches out.'

'She told me about the actual way my finger was broken and how they had fastened them together again.'

'She only told me I must keep to the diet and what I had to have and what I hadn't to have.'

In other instances the information was about more important things, but seems to have been sketchy in detail.

'That I was all right and wasn't to worry, that my progress was good and that was sweet fanny all.'

'I worried about having my womb and ovaries out, and she said, "Oh no, there's nothing wrong with them. I've seen your report. You've nothing to worry about." '

'I heard her say after the op., "Poor kid, they've only left the kitchen sink." '

So, for the 40% of patients who felt the sister gave them a little information, she seemed mainly to provide further details about something that was already basically understood, or to give rather inadequate information on more important topics.

Comments from patients who felt the sister had not given them any information again reveal patients' feelings that hospital staff often underestimate their ability to understand things: 'Personally I don't think they think that people have the intelligence to understand things.' 'She sort of just done her job. She didn't tell me anything. While I was waiting in the ante-natal ward I used to ask the sister, but she used to tell me off and said I wouldn't understand.' Others expressed doubts about the appropriate person to discuss things with: 'She thought it was the doctor's place—one seems to rely on the other.' 'I never asked. She just did her job. I got the feeling she was not supposed to discuss anyone's case.'

Other comments suggested that the sister was inaccessible 'I think she was too busy organizing the nurses to talk to the patients.' Or occasionally that she was patronizing: 'She used to come round and use this long word and say "Well, you're none the wiser are you?" and go away laughing.'

Obviously the extent to which patients feel able to discuss their problems with the sister depends on their view of her role and of her as a person. In an earlier chapter it was shown that patients were more likely to think of the sister as efficient and strict than as friendly and approachable. When asked to describe the way the ward sister looked after them, only six patients mentioned then that the sister had told them anything about their illness, treatment or progress. But when they were specifically asked later in the interview, those who said that the sister had given them a lot of information were more often enthusiastic. This can be seen in Table 20.

TABLE 20

GENERAL OPINION OF SISTER
AND INFORMATION GIVEN BY SISTER

General opinion about the way sister looked after them	Sister gave them		
	A lot of information	A little information	No information
	%	%	%
Entirely enthusiastic ..	79	69	52
Intermediate	21	28	41
Mainly critical	0	3	7
No. of patients (= 100%)	112	288	310

This suggests that some patients, at any rate, regard it as part of the sister's job to give them information. Nevertheless, half of those who had not been given any information by the sister were still enthusiastic about the way she looked after them.

Comments discussed previously suggested that it may be difficult for some sisters to combine the roles of disciplinarian and informant. They may be difficult to combine because they call for different qualities. Also patients may find it difficult to reconcile the two images—an approachable person who is easy to talk to, and one whose job is to give orders and see that they are carried out.

The Problem of Communication

The sister's role is extremely complex, involving teaching, administration, supervision and skilled practical nursing. In a ward patients are likely to see her performing all these different tasks, and to build up a picture of her as an extremely busy person, with considerable authority and responsibility. This image may give them confidence in her judgement and respect for her opinion, but may make them feel diffident about approaching her and discussing their problems with her.

The nurses

Only 4% of all the patients felt they got a lot of information about their illness, treatment or progress from the nurses, and 26% said they got a little information. The majority, 70%, said they got none.[1] Of the few patients, 11%, who said the nurses had been their main source of information, a fifth said the nurses had given them a lot of information, and the others regarded it as a little.

Examples of the type of information given by nurses suggest that it was generally straightforward, and more often about the treatment than the patient's condition.

'They explained about the stitches, those that dissolved. I was intrigued about that. They explained why you had your tummy measured—about the womb going back.'

'How long other people with the same thing had been in.'

'When they (babies) had their cords done—when it's supposed to drop off and heal up—things like that. You just talk it in conversation—it's not "I must go and ask that." '

Occasionally the nurses seemed to have phrased the information they provided in a rather unfortunate way.

'They told me how I was healing—how long it would take it to heal, and not to have intercourse until I had been seen at out-patients because it would take the scab off and undo all their work.'

Patients who said the nurses had not given them any information were asked why they thought the nurses had not done so. A few were critical.

'If you kind of probe they never say anything. It's a kind of secret weapon up there.'

'I always think you should be told what is wrong and the cause of the trouble. I asked the nurse what the pills were for. She said, "You're not supposed to know." '

[1] Question 58: 'What about the nurses, did they give you a lot of information, a little information or no information about your illness, treatment and progress? What sort of things did they tell you about?'

104

The majority justified it, in various different ways.

'They didn't like to usurp sister's job—to trespass on their seniors.'

'It's not their job to talk about what's the matter with you.'

'I didn't ask the nurses, because they don't like to speak out of turn. I'm full of admiration for them.'

'They wouldn't commit themselves. It's like in the war—we had officers above us and we had to obey orders and not give anything away.'

'They were more learners. They didn't know all that much.'

The frequency with which these types of comment occurred suggest that most of the patients did not regard the nurses as an appropriate source of information. This is confirmed by the fact that the proportion of patients who were generally enthusiastic about the way the nurses looked after them was similar among those who had and those who had not been given any information by them.

Other patients

Only 2% of the patients said that they had got most of their information about their illness, treatment and progress from the other patients, but in answer to another question 29% said they had discussed their illness or treatment together a lot, 44% that they had discussed it a little and 27% not at all.[1]

Those who had discussed their illnesses at all were asked whether they had found the discussions upsetting, and less than 1% described them as generally, 8% as sometimes, and 91% as never upsetting.[2]

Some of the few who had found the discussions upsetting appeared to have been made anxious about their own condition.

'One girl had had the op. that I was to have—it had done her no good—it was disheartening.'

Others, interpreting the question rather differently, seemed to be more concerned and distressed for the other patients.

'It was sometimes upsetting with old people who had cancer and weren't going to get better.'

'I was upset at the injustice and family tragedy of the lives of some of the chaps.'

[1] Question 79: 'Did you discuss your illnesses or treatment together a lot, a little or not at all?'
[2] Question 79 (cont.): 'Did you find these discussions at all upsetting—sometimes or generally?'

But, whereas only 9% of those who had discussed their illnesses said these discussions were upsetting, 60% said in answer to a further question that they had found them helpful.[1] Several felt that they had 'put them wise as to what to expect'.

> 'It's helpful if you're talking to a fellow who's had the same operation as you're having. You get to find out what's happening next. You're kind of more prepared for it.'

> 'Some of the fellows told me what goes on there and it helped in that respect to know what was coming.'

A number mentioned fairly specific information or advice that they had been given.

> 'I wanted more reassurance than I got from the ward sister and one of the other patients he explained to me the workings of the bowels and assured me it wasn't as necessary as I thought it was to have regular bowel movement.'

> 'I had stitches and the first time I went to the toilet it was very painful and very frightening. The other patients who had stitches explained everything to me. That's one of the things the nurses could have told me.'

Others described the reassurance, encouragement and confidence they had derived from these conversations.

> 'They put your mind at ease about things. If someone was going to have a big operation they'd say to her, "This person had it—look how well she is now." They were very good like that—very nice people in that ward.'

> 'It made you feel better when you were waiting, if there were two or three going through the same as you.'

If people are continually in wards with other patients, they are naturally curious about the illness and treatment of others, and there are likely to be discussions which some will find upsetting or embarrassing—on rare occasions even devastating. For example, one patient who had been in hospital for a mastectomy, but had not asked the surgeon what sort of growth had been removed, related how another patient came across to her and said 'Fancy you having cancer', when, she said, it had never entered her head that this was a possibility.

Only a small proportion of the patients in our sample had found the discussions at all upsetting, and a much larger proportion had found them helpful. The proportion who said they had found such discussions upsetting was highest, 17%, amongst those who said they

---

[1] Question 79 (cont.): 'Did you find them at all helpful?'

had not been able to find out all they wanted to know about their condition and treatment, and lowest, 4%, amongst those who expressed no dissatisfaction on that score. So people are less likely to be upset or distressed if they are given more adequate explanations about their own illness by the medical and nursing staff.

Summary

The discussion in the last two chapters on the various sources of information has shown how, with distant consultants, inexperienced housemen, busy and efficient sisters and uninformative nurses, the needs of the patients for information were often overlooked.

Although other patients were only rarely a major source of information, half the patients had found discussions about illnesses with other patients helpful, and less than a tenth felt they were upsetting. The proportion who were upset by them was highest among those who had been unable to find out all they wanted to know from the medical or nursing staff about their illness.

IX

IMPROVING
COMMUNICATIONS

T HE three previous chapters have discussed patients' desire for information and the difficulties they meet in obtaining it from different people. In this chapter an attempt is made to discover how communications between patients and hospital staff might be improved. It starts by considering the disadvantages of several sources of information, then looks at the relationship between patients' sources and their satisfaction with the information. Finally a suggestion is made about how some of the present difficulties might be reduced.

The disadvantages of several sources of information

Earlier it was shown that the information patients seek varies over a wide range of topics and differs in depth of detail. What is more, questions are likely to occur to patients at almost any time of the day or night while they are in hospital. It is, therefore, natural and appropriate for patients both to seek and obtain information from various sources while they are in hospital. Consultants, registrars, housemen, sisters and, to a more limited extent, nurses, all play their part in explaining things to the patients.

The main source of information of the patients in our sample is summarized in Table 21.

There is no uniformity here; no one person who is generally accepted as the most appropriate source of information. And it has been shown not only that there is variation between patients in their main source of information, but also that any patient may obtain information from several different sources.

There are a number of disadvantages in this sort of arrangement. When several people are, or may be, involved in explaining things to a patient, they will not normally be aware of what the other people have said, and explanations may be omitted, duplicated or phrased in different ways which mislead or confuse the patient or appear to him to be conflicting. An illustration of this type of misunderstanding was provided by one patient who said: 'When I went for an X-ray beforehand my own doctor told me it was to see if it was twins; the girl in hospital said it was for position; the doctor said it was to see how developed it was—so I never had a straight answer.'

When there are several possible sources the patient may not know which is the most appropriate or 'correct' person to ask, and this may increase his diffidence about asking questions.

'I wouldn't have worried so much afterwards if I'd known what they'd taken away. [Hysterectomy.] The nurses couldn't answer my questions —they're not supposed to discuss cases; and I felt in awe of the specialists and didn't ask when they came.'

'I didn't like to ask him anything. I'd rather ask sister or someone, because ,he was sort of higher. I though he mightn't like me asking details about that. I didn't know if you were supposed to ask about your condition—put it like that.'

In other instances vital pieces of information were apparently omitted and there seem to be only two possible explanations. One is that the staff were under the impression that some other member of the staff had provided it. The other likely explanation is that the

TABLE 21

MAIN SOURCE OF INFORMATION*

Informant	%
Consultant	25⎫
Registrar	6⎪ 46
House officer	12⎬
Clinical assistant	3⎭
Sister	28
Nurse	11
Other patients	2
Other source	2
No one	11
Number of patients (= 100%)	715

*This is based on the somewhat dubious assumption that the doctors whose rank could not be traced were distributed in the same way as those who could be identified.

109

information was given, but in such a way that the patient did not understand or accept it.

'I had a shock when they suddenly came to take me to the theatre. I'd already had three operations. The shock was so great I fainted. The sister was very nice about it. In fact, everyone was very apologetic, because they all thought the other one had told me.'

The multiplicity of sources, as some patients see it, gives both doctors and nursing staff an opportunity to evade questions.

'They didn't tell you anything. I didn't like asking. I'm scared stiff of doctors, but they seemed to leave it to the nurses and they didn't tell you much. They come and ask you how you are, but they don't want to listen to more. They just dash away.'

'They didn't seem to want to tell you anything. They'd put you on to someone else and to someone else. I asked the sister and one of the nurses. The nurse said, "Ask sister." Sister said, "Ask doctor", and when the specialist came he just laughed in a nice way and that was that.'

'I said to my own doctor, "Why in hospital when you ask a perfectly straightforward question do they just side-track you?" What I wanted to know was, shall I be able to carry on as I did before or shall I have to get a lighter job, and will I have a recurrence of this. The doctors wouldn't tell me anything. I asked the first in command, the second in command and they all side-tracked you. In the end they say, "Your local doctor will be informed; he'll tell you." '

The vagueness of these arrangements—the apparent lack of any clear responsibility for giving explanations—is likely to obscure from hospital staff the fact that their explanations have been inadequate, unclear or misleading, since patients will often turn to another source for clarification or elaboration.

The general practitioner, too, may find it difficult to discover what his patient has been told. One of the doctors in the sample said: 'No one has yet been designated the job of telling patients what's wrong with them.' Other general practitioners described the disadvantages of this system, or lack of system. 'If patients don't ask, the staff think someone else has told them.' 'There's always the complication that you don't know what the patient has been told. With fatal illness you've got to have some understanding between hospital doctors, nurses and the G.P. This doesn't exist at the moment.' 'Very much explaining is left to the most junior probationer nurse, who imperfectly understands the process herself.'

The evidence presented earlier showed that many patients experienced some difficulty in communicating with the hospital staff. Part of their difficulty, it is clear, arises because they are uncertain whom to turn to for information, and responsibility for this aspect of hospital care is not clearly defined. Should one person then be responsible for this, and if so, who should it be? A look at patients' sources of information and their satisfaction with it provides some guidance on this.

Satisfaction and sources

Dissatisfaction was naturally greatest among those patients who said no one had given them any information, but there were no marked differences between those whose main source of information was a doctor, a sister or a nurse, nor between those whose main informant was a consultant, registrar or house officer. This does not necessarily mean that all these groups were equally skilled or unskilled at explaining things adequately from the patient's point of view, since consultants may have been more likely to take on this task where it was particularly important or difficult. Our results indicate that each group of informants was equally successful or unsuccessful with the particular patients they informed.

The most satisfied patients were those who were given information by both the sister and the doctors. Thus, the proportions who said they were not able to find out all they wanted to know about their illness and treatment were comparatively low, 8% and 9%, in two groups: one whose main source of information was a sister but who had also found the doctors helpful, and the other group whose main source of information was a doctor, but who had also been given some information by the sister. The proportion was 23% among those whose main informant was a doctor, but who got no information from the sister, and it was also 23% among those whose main informant was the sister, but who got no information from a doctor. It was 50% among those who said they got no information from either a doctor or the sister. These figures suggest that the doctor and the sister are better viewed as partners than as alternative channels for information.

This is confirmed by the figures in Table 22, which show that patients who did not find any of the doctors helpful were comparatively unlikely to be given information by the sister.

The most probable explanation for this association is that in a hospital or department where the doctors are relatively communicative the sisters are likely to be so as well.[1] Revans[2] has shown that

---

[1] Other possible explanations are that some patients found it comparatively easy to discuss their problems with different people, or some groups of patients interpreted our questions in different ways so that they were particularly likely to regard themselves as obtaining or not obtaining information from different sources.

[2] Revans, R. W., 'Hospital attitudes and communications'.

The Problem of Communication

when the ward sister finds the people above her approachable, the nurses find the sister herself approachable. It seems likely that patients, too, will find her easier to talk to when she is able to discuss things more freely with the medical staff.

TABLE 22

INFORMATION FROM DOCTORS AND SISTER*

	Those who had found:	
	Some doctor(s) helpful	No doctor helpful
Sister gave them:	%	%
A lot of information	17	9
A little information	44	31
No information	39	60
Number of patients (= 100%) ..	553	138

* The same differences are found when medical, surgical and maternity patients are considered separately.

TABLE 23

SATISFACTION WITH INFORMATION
AND THE NURSES AND SISTER AS INFORMANTS

	Proportion not able to find out all they wanted to know	Number of patients in each group (= 100%)
Obtained information from both the sister and nurses	% 14	130
Obtained information from the sister but not the nurses ..	13	263
Obtained information from the nurses but not the sister ..	26	80
Obtained information from neither the sister nor nurses ..	33	224

Once again the nurses do not appear to play an important part in giving patients information. But, when the sister does not provide any information, they may occasionally act as a somewhat inadequate substitute. This is suggested by the figures in Table 23.

So patients' satisfaction with the information they received depended mainly on the relationship they had with both the doctors and the sister. It was important for them to be able to discuss their problems with both of them, and their satisfaction was unrelated to whether they regarded the sister or a doctor as the main informant.

A suggestion[1]

Two almost contradictory conclusions have emerged: first, that some of the difficulty in communication arises because of the multiplicity of sources of information, and second that patients who were given information by both doctors and the sister were most satisfied. This suggests that the advantages that might follow if only one member of staff gave a particular patient information might be negated because the member of staff was not there when the patient needed the information, or because of personal incompatibility.

But while the actual giving of information should not be restricted to one member of the staff, responsibility for ensuring that a patient has been given the basic information about his illness, treatment and prognosis should surely be clearly defined and should rest with one person—probably the consultant. If this were so, he would often delegate this responsibility, although ultimately it would still be his. The arrangement would thus be much the same as it is now with clinical matters, except that the form and method of delegation would be rather different here. A consultant would generally hand over this 'information' responsibility for a particular patient entirely to one member of staff—a registrar, houseman, the sister or possibly to a a staff nurse, and he would retain the responsibility himself in some instances. Who it was could depend on the circumstances and on the personalities of the particular patient and hospital staff. Occasionally it might be the general practitioner.[2] The delegation should be clear and known to all the people involved in the care of that patient—the registrar, houseman, sister and nurses—and, most important, to the patient himself. The selected staff member would make a particular point of introducing himself (or herself) to the patient, asking about any problems or queries, and telling them that if any questions arose

---

[1] A rather similar suggestion has been made independently by the Committee on 'Communication between Doctors, Nurses and Patients', which advocated the introduction of 'the concept of a personal doctor in hospital', p. 14.

[2] This is discussed in the following chapter.

they should normally ask him, but that if he was not available other members of the staff would do their best to help.

Such an arrangement need not, and indeed should not, mean that all information was provided by that one person. When other members of the staff gave or were asked for information they would let the 'chief informant' know what has happened, except when the information was of an obviously trivial nature.

Arrangements of this sort do probably exist in an informal or even unrecognized way in many hospitals or wards, but the definite adoption of such a policy might help the patients to overcome some of their very real difficulties in communicating with hospital staff. In addition it might give the members of the hospital staff more insight into these problems and could provide a very valuable part of a house officer's training, since he could undertake this responsibility in different circumstances as his experience and skill increased.

Conclusions

In this century medicine has become increasingly scientific, treatment more specific and organization more specialized. It is now frequently possible to treat and often cure diseases, where before doctors could often only hope to relieve and comfort the patients. But, in organizing the highly specialized and technical skills used in the diagnosis and treatment of illness in hospital today, the personal needs of the patients are sometimes overlooked. The physician or surgeon can call on the pathologist, the bacteriologist, the histologist and the radiologist to carry out investigations, and on physiotherapists and dieticians to help with the treatment. All these services may be admirably and efficiently organized and co-ordinated both administratively and from the clinical point of view. How does it seem to the patient? Does the person who comes to take a sample of his blood introduce himself and explain what he has come to do and why? Not invariably. Is there someone to explain this complex organization to him? Again, often there is not, and the patient has to put together scraps of information derived from different sources. Sometimes the results must be as incongruous as a game of consequences.

There appear to be several reasons for this unsatisfactory state of affairs—the diffidence of patients, the circumstances of consultation, the lack of generally accepted and clearly defined channels of communication, doctors' underestimation of patients' needs and desire for information, and their lack of skill, time, inclination and education for meeting these needs. The results are anxiety and frustration for many patients, which are not only deplorable in themselves but also lead to clinical and administrative inefficiency. As Sprott[1] puts it 'Unless there is a two-way system of communication', i.e. from patients to doctors as well as from doctors to patients, 'complaints and frustrations will pile up . . . and ultimately impair efficiency'. McGhee[2] cites, as an example of this, a patient who was given penicillin treatment, although she had warned the doctor that she had previously had a reaction. McGhee concludes that 'until the patient's need for communication is met the potentially good other aspects of his hospital care will not be fully effective'.

[1] Sprott, W. J. H., *Human Groups*, p. 123.
[2] McGhee, A., *The Patient's Attitude to Nursing Care*, pp. 50 and 76.

PART FOUR

The Hospital and the Outside World

X

THE GENERAL
PRACTITIONER AND
THE IN-PATIENT

A CONTRAST is often drawn between the impersonal care patients get in hospital—with all the problems of communication that have been described—and the more personal relationships they have with their general practitioner. It is sometimes suggested that this close relationship could continue to help patients while they are in hospital. Fox[1] puts it in this way: 'The more complex medicine becomes, the stronger are the reasons why everyone should have a personal doctor who will take continuous responsibility for him, and, knowing how he lives, will keep things in proportion— protecting him, if need be, from the zealous specialist.' And the College of General Practitioners, in a draft report on what it believes to be the content of general practice in contemporary Britain, refers to 'the family doctor's part as interpreter between his patients and consultants and specialists, hospitals, and medico-social workers'.

This chapter considers how far general practitioners fulfil this role of 'medical friend' while their patients are in hospital. It describes the contacts that patients had with their general practitioners while they were in hospital, and the attitudes of both patients and general practitioners to this relationship. The small group of patients who were under the care of their own doctor while they were in hospital are considered first.

Patients under the care of their general practitioner

Six per cent of the patients had been looked after by their own general practitioner while in hospital. A relatively high proportion of them, two-fifths, were maternity patients and there were few elderly

[1] Fox, T. F., 'The Personal Doctor and his Relation to the Hospital'.

people. As might be expected, these patients were in comparatively small hospitals—over nine-tenths were in hospitals with less than 100 beds and three-quarters in ones with 50 or less.

There was no indication that these patients were either more or less satisfied with their treatment than other patients, nor that they differed from the others in the extent to which they were satisfied with the information they had received. Some expressed appreciation of this form of medical care.

> One woman, who had been in hospital to have her first baby and whose G.P. had been present during her labour and at the birth, said, 'He's a wonderful type really, the kind you can talk to. I treated him more like my husband at the actual birth. He was wonderful, he really was.'

> Another patient, who had had a dilatation and curettage, commented: 'It was easy [to talk to the doctors], because it was my own doctor and he was very kind. He told me all I needed to know about the operation, so that I needn't ask about anything.'

Others were more critical:

> A mother, who had recently had her second baby in a maternity hospital, said: 'I hardly ever saw him [G.P.]. I don't think the doctors bother very much. Of all the doctors who came in—and there were different ones for all the girls—only one bothered to examine the girl and the baby—you know, looked to see if the stitches were O.K. and took the nappy off the baby. . . . He's not really a doctor you can talk to at all. He's moody. He's not really very attentive. He never gives you the impression he's interested.'

The numbers are, of course, small, but there is no evidence that, as is sometimes suggested, this form of medical care is especially appreciated by the patients concerned.

General practitioner visits and the attitudes of patients

Apart from those patients who had been under the care of their general practitioner, 7% had been visited by him while they were in hospital. Sometimes the contact sounded rather perfunctory and accidental:

> 'He'd been up with another patient, so he went and looked at my baby and asked how I was. There wasn't enough time to really tell him anything'.

A quarter of these patients had not discussed their illness or treatment with their doctor.[1] 'It was more of a social visit.' 'He just commiserated.' 'It was like a friend coming in.' Others had talked about

[1] Question 68: 'Did you talk to him about your illness and treatment?'

120

their illness in general terms without getting any definite information from him. 'He just asked me how I was.' 'He asked how I was getting on and said there was nothing to worry about.' 'He told me Dr. —— was very pleased with my progress.'

A third of those who had been visited by their general practitioner (2% of all patients) said they had had a helpful discussion with him about their illness.[1]

'I don't think I'd have known what had happened unless Dr. —— [G.P.] had come in during visiting time. I asked her what I'd had done. She went and read the notes and explained it all to me. Nobody else would have done.'

'The last baby had a hole in the heart and this one had his hands and feet all purple and the doctor told me it would be just the pressure, that he was all right.'

'He kept me cheerful. He was my salvation. He tried to find out about my plates. We discussed how I was feeling generally and how not to get depressed.'

But the great majority of patients, 87%, had no direct contact with their general practitioner while they were in hospital, and two-thirds of these (57% of all patients) said in answer to a direct question that they would not have liked him to visit them there.[2] Table 24 summarizes all this.

TABLE 24

CONTACTS WITH GENERAL PRACTITIONER WHILE IN HOSPITAL

	%
Looked after by G.P.	6
Visited by G.P.	
Talked about illness, discussion helpful	2 ⎫
Talked about illness, discussion not helpful	3 ⎬ 7
Did not talk about illness	2 ⎭
Not visited by G.P.	
Would have liked him to come, discussion might have been helpful	22 ⎫
Would have liked him to come, but did not think discussion about illness would have been helpful ..	8 ⎬ 87
Would not have liked him to come	57 ⎭
Number of patients (= 100%)	736

[1] Question 68 (cont.): 'Was he able to give you any helpful explanations?'
[2] Question 68 (cont.) (If doctor did not visit): (a) 'Would you have liked him to?' (b) 'Do you think it would have been helpful if you had been able to discuss your illness and treatment with him while you were in hospital?'

Most of those who did not want a visit from their general practitioner felt it unnecessary.

'I was well looked after. The vicar came.'

'I don't think there was anything he could have done more for me.'

Several people expressed the view that their doctor had plenty of other, more important, things to do.

'I had plenty of doctors—there was no need for him to waste his time.'

'I wouldn't put that on a man. He's much too overworked now.'

A few felt that he would have been superfluous.

'He's just a G.P., not a specialist.'

'I think once you go to the hospital they wipe their hands of you, say "It's not my trouble now." I've more faith in hospital than in doctors. Especially since the panel, they treat you all the same, give you the same bottle of medicine for everything.'

Other remarks suggest a superficial or somewhat unsatisfactory relationship with their general practitioner.

'There was no occasion for him to come. I don't think your panel doctors are very interested unless it's a serious case. They write out a prescription before they look at you.'

'I don't know the doctor much here. You always see someone different when you take the children down, so you never get a chance to know him.'

There were others so sceptical about the possibility of their doctor visiting them that they did not really consider it.

'He doesn't visit because of the distance. I think that's reasonable.'

'They don't usually do that, you know.'

'I'm afraid he's not the sort of doctor that would, anyhow.'

'It takes him all his time to come here (i.e. to patient's home) and he only lives over the road.'

Of those who said they would have liked their general practitioner to visit them while they were in hospital (30% of all the patients), nearly three-quarters felt it would have been helpful if they had been able to discuss their illness and treatment with him while they were in hospital. Many of these patients said they knew their general practitioner better than the hospital doctors and found it easier to talk to him.

'You can talk to your own doctor better than to strangers.'

'Your own doctor is very calming. It's the personal touch. You're not afraid to tell him what's worrying you. You get a sympathetic hearing. Others don't know you.'

There was also the feeling that on his side he would have been able to explain more readily and effectively.

'He might have told us what was really wrong.'

'He might have been able to tell me if I had cancer.'

'I felt he was the one person who would tell me what was happening.'

Patients who had earlier expressed some dissatisfaction with the information they were given while they were in hospital were more likely than the others to wish that their general practitioner had visited them. The figures are shown in Table 25.

TABLE 25

ATTITUDE TO GENERAL PRACTITIONER VISITING
AND ATTITUDE TO INFORMATION

Attitude to general practitioner visiting	*Attitude to information*		
	Not able to find out all they wanted to know	*Other difficulty in communication*	*No difficulty in communication*
	%	%	%
Would *not* have liked him to	43	63	79
Would have liked it But would not have been helpful ..	6	11	10
Would have been helpful	51	26	11
Number of patients not visited (= 100%) ..	124	253	241

The proportion who felt it would have been helpful to discuss their illness and treatment with him while they were in hospital varied from half of those who said categorically that they were not able to find out all they wanted to know to a tenth of those who reported no difficulties about this. Nevertheless, half of those with definite problems

123

either did not want their general practitioner to visit them or felt it would not have been helpful if he had done so.

When general practitioners do visit their patients, are they, in fact, able to give them the information they want? It has been shown that a third of the minority who had been visited felt they had had a helpful discussion with him, but if those who were visited are compared with those who were not, there is no difference between them in their satisfaction with the information they received. This can be seen from Table 26.

TABLE 26

ATTITUDE TO INFORMATION AND VISITS
FROM GENERAL PRACTITIONER
(Excluding patients looked after by their general practitioner)

Attitude to information	*Visited by general practitioner*	
	Yes	*No*
	%	%
Not able to find out all they wanted to know	27	20
Other difficulty in communication ..	36	41
No difficulty in communication ..	37	39
Number of patients (= 100%) ..	52	640

Further evidence that not all patients find their general practitioner particularly approachable or communicative comes from a question which asked who they found it easier to talk to, their own doctor or the doctors in the hospital;[1] 53% said their own doctor, 13% the doctors in the hospital, and 32% said there was no difference. (2% did not answer in those terms.) In spite of the difficulties of communicating with hospital doctors, which have been discussed in an earlier chapter, 45% of patients found it as easy or easier to discuss things with them as with their own doctor.

So, although 30% of patients said they would have appreciated a visit by their general practitioner, and most of these patients felt it would have been helpful to discuss their illness and treatment with him, it is doubtful whether such visits would, in fact, have helped many of them in this way.

[1] Question 109: 'Who do you find it easier to talk to—your own doctor or the doctors in the hospital?'

124

The General Practitioner and the In-Patient

When patients are not visited by their own doctor, but would like to be, how do they feel about it? Some described a sense of being abandoned.

'It would have been nice if my own doctor could have come. I'd have felt better for it. No doctor [G.P.] came at all. It's not usual now. After all, he's sent you there. If the doctor could keep in touch all the time, it would be better for you.'

'I would have liked a chat. There are some that are glad to shove you in. I think that the National Health has spoilt the doctors. They're more like clerks. Mine's good, though.'

Others felt that their general practitioner would have learnt something if he had visited them.

'If he had the time and interest to follow up my progress I think it would be helpful for him when treating future patients.'

'I think it would have given him a better understanding of the treatment I needed. It gives a better sense of continuity, you see. You get the feeling a doctor gets rid of a patient to hospital to get him off his hands and he is not too interested in him when he comes out.'

Another reaction was to feel that the hospital would not have welcomed their doctor. 'I don't think the hospital likes them coming.' 'The hospital staff doesn't like outside staff to interfere.' 'I don't think they're allowed in.'

There were other comments about the relationship between the general practitioner and the hospital doctors and the problem of responsibility.

'Of course, it's completely out of his hands once you're in another person's care.'

'I felt all these doctors are cagey about treading on each other's toes.'

'I think this much, that once your own doctor has handed you over to the specialist you can't tell him [specialist] his job. He couldn't persuade the specialist to tell me what is going on.'

There were a number of comments which suggested that patients were somewhat dissatisfied with the system of communication between the hospital and their own doctor.

'I asked about my shoulder and was told my own doctor would tell me. I would have liked to see him then.'

'If your own doctor could discuss your troubles—knowing your case history—it can be helpful for the patients and the specialist.'

'I think they should know what's going on—but I didn't tell him I was going in, so you can't altogether blame him.'

125

This last point, that their general practitioner might be unaware that they were in hospital, was made by a number of patients.

'I was told that your own doctor did visit you. But they hadn't notified my own doctor—he didn't know I'd had the baby.'

Certainly a rather higher proportion of those patients who had been admitted to hospital directly by their general practitioner had been visited than of those also referred by him but admitted from the waiting list—9% compared with 4%.

To sum up, for the great majority of patients there was no continuity of care, in the sense that they had no contact with their general practitioner while they were in hospital. Does this matter? Most of these patients either just did not expect it or would not have welcomed it, but a substantial minority, 30% of all patients, said they would have appreciated a visit from their own doctor, and most of these felt it would have been helpful to discuss their illness and treatment with him. They included a relatively high proportion of people who were dissatisfied with the information they had received while they were in hospital. But is a visit from their general practitioner the best way to solve their problems? Let us consider the views of the general practitioners on this.

Hospital visiting and the views of general practitioners

When the general practitioners in our sample were asked what they felt about visiting their patients while they were in hospital,[1] 65% felt they should do it or that they would like to do it. The main reason for this was that they felt their patients appreciated it. A fifth said that it helped to keep them informed of their patients' progress and to keep up to date with new methods of treatment, 6% welcomed the opportunity for contact with the hospital staff, and three of the doctors said it gave patients a chance to ask questions about their condition which they might not be able to put to hospital staff. Some of their comments are given below.

'It's an excellent idea. They're your patients, they just happen to be in hospital. You don't want to lose the continuity of care.'

'It's quite essential in many cases, even if you've not done anything medically, but psychologically the patients don't feel they've just been dumped.'

'It ought to be done—most important from the patient's point of view. When they go through a crisis they want to see their own doctor. It's the only way you can keep yourself informed about what's going on.'

[1] Question 22: 'What do you feel about G.P.s visiting their patients when they are in hospital?'

'It's a jolly good idea. You can see your mistakes. You get a jolly good idea of the steps by which the hospital arrives at the diagnosis. It demonstrates to the patient that you're not just a fingerpost to send them to hospital. It gives you an idea of the housemen—it's nice to know what they look like.'

Eleven per cent thought it was unwise. Most of these felt that as the clinical responsibility was no longer theirs, it would be confusing for the patients, and the hospital staff might regard it as interfering or as a nuisance.

'I'm not in favour of it at all. If they're under the hospital, it's no use two people giving opinions at once. It's unfair.'

'I do the odd visit—purely from the point of view of the patient. But I agree with some consultants that it's confusing—not a terribly sound thing on the whole. It undermines the consultant.'

'I remember vividly my own days as a houseman. It's upsetting for medical and training staff. If the G.P.'s an interfering type, it's not a good thing for the patient.'

Other reasons for regarding it as unwise were:

'In vast wards if you go in to visit one patient there may be two or four other patients of yours there, but they look quite different in hospital; you don't recognize one or two and it causes endless ill-feeling.'

'Other G.P.s think you're advertising too much.'

A further 7% felt it was just not necessary.

'It's a purely social matter. I would see any request, but it's not really necessary. They're under the care of a consultant. I have complete confidence.'

'It's a talking point. I never visit patients in hospital. It's not part of my contract. Others talk about it, but it's only their pets, or pretty girls, or fantastically interesting cases they go to see.'

And 17% did not answer in these terms, most of them saying just that there was not time or it was difficult because of the distance.

'I've not got time. Whether any useful purpose is served by going in and saying "Hello", I've grave doubts. There's no doubt patients like it.'

Altogether 16% said they did not like to appear to interfere with treatment, and that the patient was off their hands once he was admitted to hospital. Lack of time was mentioned by 38%, and distance from the hospital by 18%. Five per cent said that if one patient were visited all the others would expect it too, and 13% mentioned the difficulty of timing visits to avoid conflicting with hospital routine. Even so, nearly half felt that a visit from their general practitioner would be appreciated by patients in hospital and a third said they would like to do such visits more often.

When asked whether they thought the hospital staff welcomed, resented or felt indifferent about general practitioners visiting their patients,[1] 56% thought they welcomed them, although a quarter of these expressed certain reservations, 27% thought them indifferent, and 9% that they resented it. Eight per cent gave other answers.

Some comments were:

'The patients are delighted, the consultants quite pleased, the nurses think you're a darned nuisance.' (Welcome with qualifications.)

'You're an ordinary citizen when you go visiting a hospital. I say I've no right to probe into patients' hospital history. I'm invited and I go as a visitor.' (Other answer.)

'From my own experience they'd be apprehensive of my questioning what they were doing. There's the implication that I was checking up on what's happening to my patient, and I hate that implication.' (Resent.)

'They're pleased to see you—let me in any time. The doctors are quite prepared to let you see their notes.' (Welcome.)

'They're so surprised—they don't get over it.' (Other answer.)

When they were asked to estimate the number of patients they had visited in hospital in the last twelve months a quarter of them said they had not visited any, and another quarter that they had visited less than 10. At the other end of the scale, a fifth said they had seen on average at least one a week, or 50 or more during the course of a year.

However, if general practitioners are to visit their patients in hospital they need to know when they have been admitted. Only four out of the 124 general practitioners said they were generally informed by the hospital when their patients had been or were about to be admitted from the waiting list.[2] Some felt it would be helpful if they were told.

'I would like it. It's awkward when you call to visit and find a person's been admitted.'

'Yes, I would like it, otherwise you keep wondering if they're going to blow up with an appendix.'

[1] Question 25: 'When you go, do you feel the hospital staff welcome your visit, resent it or are indifferent?'
[2] Question 12: 'Do you generally know when a patient has been or is about to be admitted—in time to visit him in hospital if you wanted to?—Always or generally? Who do you hear this from most often?'

The General Practitioner and the In-Patient

'It's a bit awkward when you ask a patient if they've had their operation and they say "Oh, yes—didn't you know?" You look a bit silly.'

'Very often you don't know they're in until you hear from the relations, casually. It would help a lot to know, but the general impression at —— hospital is that the G.P. either doesn't exist or else he's an awkward thing that's got to be co-operated with.'

Several of them said that the patients themselves or their relatives would usually let them know, and the majority seemed to accept this somewhat haphazard arrangement uncritically. A number said they did not want or need such information.

'I'm not sure that's necessary. There's enough paper work as it is. Gone is the day when you visit your hospital patients.'

'I generally hear through the grapevine. It would be nice [to be notified] but it wouldn't make any difference—it's not worth it.'

'I haven't time to visit. Once a patient is in hospital I'm inclined to dismiss him from my mind—write him off.'

Others felt it was up to the patient to let them know.

'I don't see why patients shouldn't inform us themselves—to save the hospital. They usually assume that you know. Patients think you know everything.'

'It's up to the patient—he should inform his doctor. But I'm not particularly interested in visiting.'

It seems therefore that few patients are visited in hospital by their general practitioners, partly because doctors find it difficult to make the time to do this and partly because they feel it unnecessary or unwise. Do general practitioners, then, feel that their patients do not need their aid while they are in hospital? Seventy-one per cent said, in answer to a direct question, that they did not feel that hospitals kept patients reasonably informed about their illness and treatment.[1] A further 19% were doubtful and only 10% were apparently happy about this aspect of hospital care. Some were emphatically critical:

'It's my *bête noire*. The vast majority of information patients get in hospital is from overheard conversations which in many cases don't even concern that patient.'

'No. Patients come out completely ignorant. They haven't a clue and only one in ten will ask. Hospital doctors are notorious for not letting them know anything. You have to explain yourself. It's often a tremendous relief to them when you do.'

[1] Question 30: 'Do you think hospitals keep patients reasonably informed about their illnesses, and the treatment they receive?'

Several mentioned that patients often did not know what had been done at an operation.

'Many patients try to get information and can't. Many a patient goes to the operating theatre without knowing why.'

'No—they haven't a clue what they've had done to them. It's amazing. It's remarkable how many ask me what's been done in a surgical operation.'

'Often people come out and don't know what they've had done—even what operations they've had. They expect us to tell them and often we don't get enough information either.'

The patients' ignorance was explained in various ways.

'A lot are not informed at all and others misinterpret it. They're nervous and don't take in what's said.'

'I imagine the reason is that several people are looking after a patient. They all think the others are going to do it.'

'Consultants are not prepared to spend five minutes talking to patients, discussing their illness.'

'Patients almost invariably say they're not told anything. I believe this is almost entirely because of their inability to grasp what they've been told.'

They were asked whether they thought that—given a closer contact between general practitioners and hospitals—the general practitioners could do more to keep hospital patients informed, or whether they thought hospitals should improve their handling of this on their own.[1] Most of those who were at all critical of the way hospitals kept patients informed—and 46% of all the general practitioners—thought that the hospital should improve on its own.

'You don't want to have men on the bridge while the patient's in hospital. The consultant's in charge; he should decide what to tell, and should tell the G.P.s what he has told. If the G.P. was brought in, he might put his foot in it and get under sister's feet. It's possible that patients are not told enough. Certainly some of the things they say they've had done are very peculiar—but then there are some very peculiar surgeons these days.'

'I think it's up to the house surgeon. They should treat patients as people, not as cases—they give the impression of treating them as cases. If

[1] Question 31: 'If there was a closer or more intimate contact between G.P.s and hospitals, do you think G.P.s could help to keep hospital patients better informed about things—or do you think there is little room for improvement, or do you think hospitals should improve their way of handling this on their own?'

they were treated as people, surely they'd be told enough to help them along. That's the mistake of going through training and then straight into hospital. They never see patients at home.'

'While in hospital, when they're under tension, that's when they're most worried—that's the time they want to know.'

Seventeen per cent thought the general practitioner should help with this.

'The G.P. must decide with his knowledge how much the patient should be told and how he should be told. The information doesn't come quickly enough. Patients build up the idea that you're stalling when you say you haven't heard.'

'They're our patients and we know them better. It's the hospital's job to treat them, our job to explain things. Patients go into hospital to get better. If they do, I don't see it matters much [explaining things]. Before N.H.S. only patients with a low income went into hospital, and nothing was explained.'

And 19% thought that not only should the hospitals improve their handling of this but that the general practitioners could help, too.

'Where possible the G.P. should inform the patient. Patients look to the G.P. as a friend and the consultant as a demi-god. But the G.P. and the consultant must give the same story. I had told a patient with cancer of the uterus there was no cure for her and she had accepted it. When the consultant saw her in hospital on admission for an emergency op. he told her that she'd be all right. This mustn't happen. I think G.P.s have a big role to play in helping those for whom there is no cure.'

'It's best to do it through the patient's own doctor, but it's a good thing if they can give them some sort of inkling.'

'Some patients do things for consultants because of discipline, others do it if you know them. In hospital they lack confidence in themselves— they ask us questions which they wouldn't dream of asking in hospital.'

Finally, 18% thought there was no need for improvement. Some of their comments suggest that they may not have very high expectations.

'The hospitals very often leave it to us and then we do it if necessary. It works all right. Most people you can't explain things to. If they've no knowledge of anatomy and physiology you can't explain, no matter how intelligent they are.'

'As far as I know there's no need for improvement. I don't mean to say the patient should know every little thing—like a drug, what it's for. If they say "You've got a bad heart and I'm going to treat it", that's enough. It's no business of his how they're going to treat it.'

'Provided they [hospital] let us know the facts, we can explain afterwards. Patients may suffer unnecessary anxiety temporarily.'

131

Most of the general practitioners, though, were well aware that patients often leave hospital ignorant about what has been done to them, bewildered and anxious about the implications of their illness. Many of them felt that the responsibility for this rests entirely with the hospital; others that general practitioners could or should do something to help. Among the latter were some who thought that the general practitioner should be involved in this during the patient's stay in hospital and others who felt that full explanations from the general practitioner could be left until the patient is out of hospital.

At present even the few visits made by general practitioners to patients in hospital do not seem to do much to resolve the patients' problems of communication. So, if the general practitioner is to be really effective here, a more satisfactory procedure would be needed, and his role and responsibilities clearly defined. Such an arrangement is probably particularly appropriate for patients with a serious[1] or fatal illness who know their general practitioner well and have a reasonably close relationship with him. For others with minor conditions, and for those who have had little contact with their general practitioner and do not have a particularly personal relationship with him, such an arrangement is not necessarily an advantage. Certainly if general practitioners were normally to take on this responsibility it would demand radical changes in the habits and outlook of most of them, and in hospital procedures and organization.

On the other hand, if patients were given only minimal or basic explanations while they were in hospital, and it was left to the general practitioners to provide fuller explanations after they had come out, this would have other disadvantages. The major one is that patients would have to wait for full explanations. This would surely be unfortunate. Patients should not be left to guess, worry and surmise about what is the matter with them, what is being done about it and how it will affect them. What is to be done at an operation, for instance, should be explained beforehand and confirmed immediately afterwards. Because of this, it seems unlikely that such a policy would be generally acceptable to hospital staff. There is also the problem of the interpretation of 'minimal or basic' information, and the difficulty that there is often some delay before the general practitioners themselves receive the information from the hospital. Over a third of the doctors in our sample complained of the length of time they waited to receive a full report after discharge, and 12%

---

[1] 'Serious' here is not intended to be confined to illnesses which are dangerous to life, but to include any illness likely to have a considerable effect on the patient's life or outlook, such as incapacitating illness, conditions which are likely to prevent patients continuing in the same type of work, and conditions and operations which affect their reproductive functions.

complained of the lack of a prompt discharge note.[1] There was also some criticism of the amount of information they received.[2]

Summary and conclusions

Many general practitioners have mixed feelings about visiting their patients in hospital and few do it at all frequently, although many feel that their patients would appreciate visits. Time and distance are important deterrents, but there also appears to be some ambiguity about their relationship with their patients while they are in hospital. Some general practitioners will look at their patient's medical notes and discuss things with the patients and with the hospital medical staff. Others regard themselves purely as visitors and feel that any discussion of their patients' illness or treatment would be an unwarranted interference in what should be entirely the consultant's responsibility. When discussing the way in which hospitals kept patients informed about their treatment and progress, most general practitioners felt there was room for improvement and, while just over half of these felt it was up to the hospital to improve their own arrangements, just under half felt that the general practitioners could or should help with this. There is thus a wide difference of opinion among the general practitioners themselves about the task of keeping hospital patients informed about their condition, treatment and progress.

This variation in the views and habits of the general practitioners may partly account for the present unsatisfactory arrangements made by many hospitals. As long as there is any ambiguity, responsibility for what is a difficult and time-consuming job can more readily be shelved.

Here again clarification is needed, and it is suggested that the responsibility must rest with the hospital staff, but that arrangements should be made for this responsibility to be clearly handed over to the general practitioner when he feels it is desirable. Unless or until the general practitioner formally states that he wishes to accept this responsibility for a particular patient, it should rest with the consultant or the person to whom he delegates it. When a general practitioner has undertaken this, he will need to visit the patient in hospital and also to discuss the position with the staff there. It is also

[1] Question 8: 'What do you feel about the ways in which hospitals keep G.P.s informed about their patients' progress and the treatment and investigation which is being carried out?' Question 11: 'Do you feel you generally receive the information soon enough?'

[2] Fifty-one per cent said they were *always* given enough information, 39% that they *usually* had enough and 10% that they did not generally get enough. (Question 7.)

necessary for the hospitals and the general practitioners to keep each other informed not only of the investigations and treatment they have carried out, but also of the explanations they have given to patients. Occasionally hospitals do make provisions for this on the form they send out, but this ought to be the rule and not the exception.

At the moment, however, when few patients are visited by their general practitioner and many feel they have been given inadequate explanations by the hospital staff, one must agree with McKeown[1] 'that the personal service is far from satisfactory in Great Britain today, because it is virtually restricted to the domiciliary scene and breaks down . . . when the patient enters hospital'.

[1] McKeown, T., 'The Future of Medical Practice outside the Hospital'.

XI

FAMILIES AND FRIENDS

M ost patients are only in hospital for a short while. Their stay is a temporary break in their normal lives, and even while they are away from home they are, of course, still members of a family. The various ways in which relatives and neighbours help the patient and his immediate family are described in this chapter. It begins by seeing how far patients were isolated from their family and friends while they were in hospital, and also looks at the difficulties of people who live alone.

Visiting

Although other patients are often a source of companionship and support, contact with their own family and friends is obviously of great importance to people who are ill and living in a strange environment. Visiting times are eagerly awaited. 'You used to be looking forward to that all day.' 'You don't feel so bad if you see someone every night.'

Opportunities for visiting have in general increased in recent years and most of the patients in our sample, 88%, could have visitors every day. It is still usual, however, for visiting to be confined to a limited period, often only half an hour on most days, and for the numbers of visitors to be restricted. When asked what they thought about the visiting hours and arrangements,[1] 30% of the patients expressed unqualified approval, a similar proportion found them 'satisfactory' or 'all right', 15% voiced some qualifications with their approval, and 22% were mainly critical.[2]

Several patients, 17%, expressed appreciation of the frequency with which they could have visitors. 'It was wonderful just to see my husband every night.' Others, 16%, praised the flexibility shown by the hospital staff.

[1] Question 24: 'What did you think of the visiting hours and arrangements?'
[2] The others expressed both praise and criticism.

'Mother is very old and could only come to see me when there was someone to bring her. The hospital let her come in, at odd times—whenever she could, they were very considerate.'

'If your visitors couldn't come at the right time they arranged another time for them. They were really very good about that.'

'I thought it was wonderful. They had a long time for visitors and didn't chase them away.'

Latitude over the number of visitors allowed was also appreciated.

'I thought they were grand. There was never anyone turned away no matter how many were around the bed.'

'There was only supposed to be one visitor, being the maternity ward, but they never sort of turned them out or said anything about it. I used to have about three.'

But a number of patients had found the hospital staff less accommodating.

'Only thing if Jack came, mother couldn't. They couldn't change over, as in some hospitals.'

'They're clock watching for throwing-out time—visitors appear to be looked on as a necessary menace.'

This kind of rigidity was particularly frustrating when visitors found the times inconvenient.

'I think the hours should be extended for those who have to rush home, like my husband. If he missed the bus he was 15 minutes late.'

'It was difficult, because my husband's not home by that time and he couldn't always get there with putting the baby to bed. I did ask the Sister the first time, but she said, "No, not out of hours." '

'You could come every night, but my husband couldn't come at the right time, so they wouldn't let him in.'

Altogether 12% said the visiting hours were inconvenient, and 17% felt they were too short.

'The clock used to go on wheels; before you knew where you were it was over. That half-hour looked about 10 minutes. Only just a few words lift you up a little.'

'I think it might be an hour in the evenings instead of half an hour. People at work all day rush up there—by the time they get to the top of the stairs it's time to come back again.'

Several patients mentioned the distance that their friends and relatives had to travel, and the expense that this entailed.

'It was too short for the distance people have to travel. It's all right for them as lives near, but not for others.'

'The time was too short. It was only half an hour, but the journey took two hours.'

'Well, it's a long way to come for half an hour and I used to tell him [husband of 83] he mustn't come on any account except for the hour—that was Wednesdays and Sundays.' (Half an hour other days.)

Because of this some patients would have preferred less frequent longer, visits.

'Half an hour every night, an hour on Sundays. It's not very long for people that have to come a distance. It ought to be longer and not so frequent.'

This problem is likely to increase as the district general hospitals envisaged under the Hospital Plan[1] are developed, and replace small local hospitals.

The patients themselves seemed to prefer evening visiting, as well as finding it more convenient for their visitors.

'Everything seems to go dead when they've gone. All the patients seem to draw into themselves and just lie quiet. It's different in the evenings, when the nurses have to start getting ready for lights out.'

'If it was afternoons the evening dragged, but if it was evenings you look forward to visitors during the afternoons.'

'Everybody remarked that they didn't like the afternoon visiting; it made the evenings too long, even though you had the TV and radio.'

One aspect of visiting arrangements which unfortunately we did not ask about specifically was whether children could visit. A number of patients said spontaneously that they wished their children could have come.

'You miss your children more than your husband. The boy of 14 came, but the young one wasn't allowed.'

'You can't bring babies into the ward and I missed my little girl.'

'I do think you should be allowed to see your children when you are in. My little girl lost her sleep through missing me.'

'I fretted like mad for the kids.'

One or two mentioned that it had been possible to arrange it, and they had obviously appreciated it greatly.

'I had the children up over Christmas. I was thrilled to see them.'

[1] *A Hospital Plan for England and Wales*, op. cit.

137

The Hospital and the Outside World

Many hospitals now recognize the distress that children in hospital feel when they are separated from their parents, but obviously children whose parents are in hospital are also likely to feel deprived. Of the women in our sample, a third left a dependent child under 15 at home when she went into hospital, and a fifth a child who was under 5. Nearly half of those with young children under 5 were maternity patients, two-fifths were surgical patients and a tenth medical.

If unrestricted visiting was allowed over a large part of each day this would overcome the difficulty of inconvenient times. It is also likely that if visiting times were less formal there would be less pressure on relatives to come every time. Certainly the present arrangements in many hospitals, with visiting for short fixed times every day, must impose a burden on many relatives who may also have extra responsibilities at home while the patient is in hospital. A number of the patients in our sample were well aware of this.

'I would have liked it less [frequently] because people had so far to come, but the family were always there, although I told them not to.' (Visiting every day.)

'Too much really. If someone can go every night they feel they *must* go, and it costs a lot.'

'I think there's too many [visiting times], between you and me and the gate post. It drags the wife out every day when she could be having a rest. It's very acceptable for the patient, but you've got to think of the other people.'

And formal visiting times can create a feeling of strain and artificiality.

'It seemed to fly over. I used to get palpitations when the time came for them to go.'

'I would like a bit more privacy—draw the curtains round or something. It was all a bit embarrassing and my husband used to get so confused that it spoilt it—just an anti-climax really, when you've been looking forward to it all day.'

If visiting was more staggered, some patients might be able to see their visitors in side rooms or sitting-rooms in a more private and intimate atmosphere. And if there were no formal visiting times it would be less distressing for the patient with no visitors. At the moment, as one put it, 'It's not so good when you don't have visitors.'

One of the main arguments against unrestricted visiting is that it would disrupt the hospital routine. Comments from a number of patients show that formal arrangements do not always avoid this:

'One thing that I thought was queer was the matron and sister came round to ask how you were when the visitors were there.'

'The doctors used to come round just on visiting time and that cut the visiting time short. I did feel they could have arranged that a bit better.'

'Every evening visiting from 7 to 7.30 and the evening meal was at 7.10. In that half-hour you can't eat and talk to your visitors at the same time!'

With sudden emergencies it may, in fact, be more difficult for the hospital staff to clear the ward during fixed visiting hours than it would be for them with unrestricted visiting times. Fewer visitors would be there at any one time, and they would be more likely to understand and accept the temporary closing of the ward if they knew they could come back later when the crisis was over.

One study[1] of the habits and attitudes of visitors and nursing staff before and after the introduction of free visiting in the geriatric wards of an acute general hospital found that free visiting was preferred by the nurses and led to greater co-operation between hospital staff and visitors.

Another argument put forward against it is that patients would find unrestricted visiting too tiring, but the sister in a ward could obviously, at her discretion, restrict either the length of time or the number of visitors allowed for particular patients. The present usual system which fixes these for all patients, often irrespective of how they feel, is likely to be a strain on some patients while frustrating others. 'When you're feeling ill the hour seemed too long, but as soon as you're feeling better it goes by—whoosh!' As it was, one or two felt they had been allowed visitors when they would have been better without them.

'The night of my op. my husband came, but it's not wise to have visitors, because you don't know anything. One woman, she told her husband to go away—you know people are sick and they don't mean it, but it hurts just the same.'

The Minister of Health has recently asked all hospitals to experiment with more liberal arrangements such as unrestricted daily visiting between 2 p.m. and 8 p.m.[2] Although some hospitals have introduced effective schemes, others have been less successful, and it seems that such arrangements need careful introduction to relatives, patients, and possibly most important of all, the nursing staff.

Patients' desire for frequent contact with their families and friends was generally recognized by their relatives. Three-quarters of the

---

[1] Irvine, R. E., and Smith, B. J., 'Patterns of Visiting'.
[2] Ministry of Health, *Circular on Visiting of Patients*.

patients in hospitals with daily visiting times had visitors on every possible occasion. This can impose a burden on relatives in both time and expense at a time when they may have extra jobs to do at home, such as housework and looking after children if the patient is a housewife and a mother. Fixed visiting times add to the difficulty of arranging for the care of children and making the most of travelling facilities, and when the time of the visit is short, the journey may seem less worth while, but relatives may feel they must take extra care to arrive punctually so that none of the precious time together is lost. If visiting times were generally less restricted, friends and relatives could visit when it was most convenient for them.

Fathers

Apart from normal visiting, maternity patients may also want company and support during labour. Three-fifths of the maternity patients were left alone at some stage during their labour and nearly a third of them felt critical or resentful about this.[1] When they were asked if there was anyone else they would have liked to be there, the person most frequently mentioned was their husband, but nearly as many patients wanted more medical or nursing staff with them at that time.[2] Nineteen per cent of the patients said that their husbands were with them at some time during the early stages of labour, although none were present for the actual birth, but when asked directly another 16% said they would have liked him to be there.[3]

This issue—whether or not husbands can be present during labour—seems worthy of special examination. First, here are the remarks of two wives who wanted their husbands to be there:

'As he wanted to, I would have liked him to have stayed. Some of the other husbands made a fuss and stayed, but I think the staff made the wife suffer because they had.'

'I think when you are very much in love with your husband it gives you lots of confidence. He does give me confidence and helps me.'

Sometimes the patient had never asked if it could be arranged.

'I never made inquiries. I don't think they like it.'

Others had asked and found it not possible.

'I'd have liked my husband to be there. He came for half an hour in the night, but they sent him away.'

---

[1] Question 35: 'Were you left alone at all before the baby was born?' Question 36: 'How did you feel about that?'
[2] Question 37: 'Who was with you mainly?' Question 38: 'Is there anyone else you would have liked to be there?'
[3] Question 39: 'Was your husband with you at all—in the early stages—when the baby was born?' 'Would you have liked him to be there?'

'I would have loved him to be there—that was why I would have liked it at home, but unfortunately I couldn't. No, they don't allow it.'

But the majority, two-thirds, said they would not have liked their husbands to be with them. A number of them felt it was not suitable or appropriate for men.

'I would have liked his comfort, but not for him to see me like that in pain. He can't bear to see anybody he loves in pain. He said he didn't realize what a woman had to go through.'

'If the men were with you, there'd never be any more. I wouldn't like my husband round there, in any case.'

'I think it's a job you have to get on with yourself. It's embarrassing enough with strange women there, let alone a man.'

'I didn't want him there. The further away the better. I'm afraid when you're in a bit of pain you don't have a good word for the husbands.'

Some of those who did not want their husband to be present wanted him to be near at hand.

'I wouldn't like him to be there at the birth. I'd be a bit self-conscious—it might put him off. He was in the corridor and the doctor held her up before she was washed or anything for him to see—which I thought was nice.'

'I wouldn't want him with me actually—I would have just been content to know he was there, but they wouldn't allow him to stay, although it was only a matter of an hour and a half before the baby was born. It would have saved him worrying, going home and phoning the hospital afterwards.'

'They were very good. As soon as the baby came, before they cleaned me or the baby up, they let him into the theatre to see me. I was a bit muzzy, but it was nice to know he'd been there.'

So, although many women said they did not want their husband to be with them while their baby was born, a number would have liked it, and others would have appreciated his presence during the early stages of labour or soon after the baby was born. Moreover, the proportion who would like their husbands to be there is likely to increase in the future. None of the women in our sample who were aged 35 or more wanted this, but a fifth of the younger mothers did. (Table 27.)

At present facilities are often inadequate for the minority of couples who would like to be together, and there is some evidence that hospital staff are not always sympathetic to their wishes. But some wives would derive confidence and comfort from the presence of their husbands if it could be arranged.

TABLE 27

VARIATIONS WITH AGE IN ATTITUDE
TO HUSBAND'S PRESENCE DURING LABOUR

(Maternity patients only)

	Wife's age	
	Under 35	*35 or more*
	%	%
Husband present during early stages ..	22	5
Husband not present:		
Would have liked him to be there ..	20	—
Would *not* have liked him to be there	58	95
Number of patients (= 100%) ..	91	22

How the family manages while the housewife is in hospital

As well as visiting the patient while he or she is in hospital, the families[1] of patients who are housewives and mothers have the additional problem of coping with housework and looking after children.

Two-thirds of these families had had some help from relatives, neighbours or friends while the housewife was in hospital.[2] With 40% it was the housewife's relatives who helped, and with 17% her husband's; demonstrating once again the strength of the ties between the women in a family.[3] Fourteen per cent of the families had been helped by friends or neighbours and only 1% by a home help. So in this kind of crisis ties of kinship and friendship are of much greater importance than official sources.

The kind of help given differed widely. Neighbours shopped and lit fires, sisters did the washing and had husbands in for meals, married daughters cooked, nieces cleaned and various people helped with looking after the children. When mothers of children under 15 went into hospital, the children went to stay with relatives in 27% of the families, and in 29% relatives not normally living in the house

[1] This is used here loosely to cover people who are related and living in the same household.

[2] Question 104; 'While you were in hospital did anyone have time off work or school to do things in the house? Did they have any help from anyone not living here? What about your own relatives, in-laws, neighbours, home help, or anyone else?'

[3] See also Young, M., and Willmott, P., *Family and Kinship in East London*; and Willmott, P., and Young, M., *Family and Class in a London Suburb*.

142

helped to look after them. Sometimes relatives came from other districts and lived in the household. Other families had relatives living nearby who could come round during the day or to whom the children could go for their tea when they came out of school. Neighbours or friends helped look after the children in another 14% of families, 4% had help from various other sources, and 26% managed without much help.

'He had his lunch at school and his dad gave him tea at night and got him up in the morning.'

'The children went to school as usual after their father had given them breakfast. They stayed for meals at school, then they came to hospital with him and waited or stayed at home and watched the telly.'

It is not possible to assess how satisfactory these arrangements were. Some patients were worried and anxious about what was happening at home.

'The thing I was really worried about when I was rushed away for the emergency was there was no one to look after the children. I haven't got any parents and my husband's a long-distance lorry driver. They might fix something about that. It really pulls you down, that worry.'

Sometimes relatives had stayed off work to do housework or look after the children. This happened in 14% of all households when the patient was the housewife, and in 19% of these households with children. In two-thirds of these instances money was lost as a result, but with the others the time off was taken as paid holiday. Occasionally it was the husband or father who stayed off work, but daughters, mothers and sisters also did, and it may well be that women are more likely to be expected to stay away from work on these occasions than men.

In 2% of the housewives' families a child had had time off school and this proportion was 6% in households with schoolchildren. Seven of the eight children were girls.

Two mothers had got into trouble over this.

'I had to keep her (Sarah, aged 14) home to look after Susan. I was fined £2 for that, for her not being at school, but they won't get that. Sarah's very good, though. She can cook and do all the housework and so on.'

'We had a bit of trouble over that. She was off one day for the washing and late every morning to clear up. My husband phoned the head-mistress and told her she was going to take time off.'

Coming home

The families' difficulties do not always cease when the patient comes out of hospital. He or she may need looking after when they come home, and if the patient is a housewife it may be some time before she can take up her normal household tasks.

When they left hospital the majority of patients, 87%, went back home immediately, 5% went to a convalescent home, 7% went to stay with relatives and 1% had other arrangements. People living on their own much more often went to a convalescent home or to stay with relatives, but three-fifths even of them went straight back to their own home. Among the others, women were more likely than men to go to stay with relatives, but no more likely to go to a convalescent home. These variations are shown in Table 28.

TABLE 28

WHERE PATIENTS WENT AFTER LEAVING HOSPITAL
AND THEIR POSITION IN THE HOUSEHOLD

(Excluding patients still in hospital)

	Position in household				
	Lives alone	*Male head of household*	*Female head of household*	*Female housewife*	*Other*
	%	%	%	%	%
Straight to own home	61	94	83	86	90
Convalescent home	19	5	3	4	2
To relatives ..	17	1	11	9	2
Other	3	—	3	1	6
Number of patients (= 100%) ..	59	223	29	353	50

Most patients, 85%, felt they had been discharged at the right time, 8% felt it was too soon and 7% thought they could have come home earlier.[1] In making this estimate they were asked to consider both their health and their home circumstances, but of course their ideas may not always have been realistic.

A number of those who felt they had come out too early referred to the pressure on hospital beds.

[1] Question 102: 'Did you feel you were discharged from hospital too soon, about the right time, or do you feel you could have come out earlier—considering both your illness and home circumstances?'

144

'They're in a hurry to get rid of you'. (In hospital less than two weeks for removal of breast with malignant growth.)

'They sent me out on a stretcher. You're rarely in for 10 days, because of the shortage of beds. They go in and out like a cattle market.' (In hospital less than a week. Maternity patient.)

'I got my stitches out and came straight home. It was because of the shortage of beds. The wound was still discharging and my husband had to dress it.' (In hospital for between three weeks and a month for mastectomy.)

On the other hand, some of those who felt they could have come out earlier described their frustration when nothing much seemed to be happening.

'I felt fit three days before, but I had to wait until the doctor came on the Monday.'

'It was Easter-time and the staff were on holiday. I had to wait for the X-ray.'

'You have to wait for the doctor. Perhaps there's something wrong with the works—people get brought in and forgotten. There's a lot of marking time, but they may have definite reasons for this.'

Others had been anxious to get home to their families. 'My daughter was taking advanced G.C.E. I felt I was getting on all right and wanted to come home to be with her for it'.

What happened when the patients got home? All the housewives, including those living on their own, were asked about extra help they had, after they got home, with shopping, cooking, cleaning, washing or looking after children.[1] Thirty-seven per cent of housewives had received some help from relatives not living in the household, 33% from other people in the same household, 11% from friends and neighbours, 4% from a home help and 5% from other sources. Of the 30% who had not received any extra help, a third said they could have done with some.

Once again relatives are the most frequent source of help, but inevitably this form of help acts in a somewhat 'arbitrary' manner, not being directly related to need. To some extent those with the heaviest responsibilities—with young children or old people to look after—are rather less likely to get help from relatives outside the household than other housewives. (Table 29.)

All patients, not only housewives, were asked whether they had had any help since they left hospital from a district nurse, health

---

[1] Question 105: 'When you got home did you have any more help than usual with the shopping, cooking, cleaning, washing or looking after children?' IF YES, 'Who helped?' IF NO, 'Could you have done with some?'

TABLE 29

SOURCE OF HELP AFTER RETURN HOME
FOR HOUSEWIVES WITH VARYING RESPONSIBILITIES

(Housewives only, excluding those still in hospital)

	With children under 10*	With children aged under 15, but none under 10	With adults aged 65 or more†	With adults aged 15 to 64 only
	%	%	%	%
Received help from:				
Relatives not in household ..	33	43	27	43
Friends and neighbours ..	13	13	16	7
Home help ..	3	8	4	1
Others	6	5	2	3
No help outside household	51	40	51	48
Number of patients (= 100%)	120	40	45	164

* With or without older children.
† Without children.

visitor, home help, or similar person.[1] Nine per cent had help from a health visitor, 8% from a district nurse, 3% from a home help and 1% from a midwife.

Among the 81% who had no help from these sources were 7% who said they would have liked a home help. But to a number of housewives the idea of a stranger coming into their homes to do housework was abhorrent.

'I don't want strangers. We're the kind of family that help each other. My daughter did the house and the cooking and that.'

'I didn't want a home help. They know too much about your private affairs—not that we've anything to be ashamed of.'

'I wouldn't like to have a lady in the place—it's a bit rough.'

[1] Question 106: 'Have you had any help from a district nurse, home help, health visitor or anyone like that since you left hospital?' IF NO, 'Do you think any of those people could have helped you?'

146

Others who felt it would have been helpful had been deterred from making inquiries about the possibility by the thought of the cost.

'I didn't think about it at the time. We're not in a position to afford a home help, anyway, but it would have been a help, cleaning the house and keeping it tidy.'

'I could have done with a home help, but they want you to pay for them and when you're on a pension you can't afford it.'

People who lived on their own were more likely than other housewives to have had a home help, but since this form of help is much less common than help from other sources, nearly half of those living on·their own had no help at all with the housework when they came home, compared with about a quarter of other housewives. They were if anything rather less likely than other housewives to be helped by relatives outside the household and they were no more likely than others to be given help by friends and neighbours. These differences are shown in Table 30.

TABLE 30

SOURCE OF HELP AFTER RETURN
FOR PEOPLE LIVING ALONE AND OTHER HOUSEWIVES

(Housewives only, excluding those still in hospital)

	Living on own	Other housewives
	%	%
Received help from:		
Relatives—not in household ..	24	38
Friends and neighbours ..	10	11
Home help	14	3
Others	12	4
Others in same household only	—	38
No help		
Could have done with some ..	16⎫48	8⎫27
Did not need any	32⎭	19⎭
Number of patients (= 100%) ..	50	369

Thus, although people who lived alone were more likely to go to a convalescent home or to have a home help, several of them still had difficulty in managing when they first came home after a spell in hospital. Who were these people, and what other problems did they have in connexion with a stay in hospital?

The Hospital and the Outside World

People who live alone

The most notable way in which they differed from other patients was in their age. Sixty-five per cent were over 65, compared with 13% of other patients. Put in another way, 38% of the older patients aged 65 or more lived on their own, compared with 4% of other patients. Another difference, associated with this but not so marked, was that a relatively high proportion were women, 76% against 62% of other patients.

There is some evidence from this survey that people living on their own were kept in hospital rather longer than others. Among women of 65 or more, half of those living alone stayed in hospital for a month or more, compared with a fifth of those living with other people. This difference could not be explained by other variations in the two groups. The proportion of surgical patients was similar, 36% of those living alone and 40% of others, and the proportion aged 75 or more was only slightly greater among those living alone, 44% compared with 36%, a difference which might well have occurred by chance. So the length of time patients were kept in hospital appears to be related not only to their illness and treatment but also to the social conditions in which they were living.

It is widely recognized that hospitals are sometimes reluctant to admit elderly people because of the difficulty in finding somewhere for them to go when they are fit to leave hospital, and it is possible that elderly people living on their own may be at an even greater disadvantage in this respect than those living with friends or relatives. The numbers in our survey are too small to produce any definite evidence here. But there is no doubt that, when they are taken ill or have an accident, there may be some delay before anyone else realizes this or does anything about it. The stories of two patients illustrate this.

A widow in her seventies broke her thigh when she fell off a chair in her kitchen. She described how she had to crawl to the front door and call out. 'Finally people heard me, but they could not get in. Two policemen came past; they put a little girl through the window and she opened the door. It's terrible when you live alone. I was lying like that from two o'clock till four in the afternoon.'

A woman in her sixties whose husband had died recently, was taken ill with a bad cold and chest. 'I was in an awful state. I went to our doctor, was given a bottle of medicine and some tablets and told to go to bed for a couple of days.' A neighbour called the doctor in a week later when she came in and found her so ill. The doctor then got her admitted straight away—with double pneumonia and pleurisy.

So even when people do get into touch with their doctor initially, if they live on their own it may be difficult to reach him again later. Elderly people living alone are the ones least likely to have a telephone. Only 5% of people aged 65 or more and living on their own had a telephone, compared with 23% of other people of this age and 21% in the sample as a whole.

As might be expected, too, people living alone had fewer visitors than others while they were in hospital. (Table 31.)

TABLE 31

FREQUENCY WITH WHICH VISITED
BY AGE AND WHETHER LIVING ALONE

	Under 65		65 or more	
	Living alone	*Not living alone*	*Living alone*	*Not living alone*
Had visitors:	%	%	%	%
Every visiting time	41	78	45	68
Most visiting times	27	16	37	26
Less frequently	32	6	18	6
Number of patients (= 100%)	22	560	38	85

When they were at home, how isolated were those living alone? Twenty-five per cent had relatives whom they saw every day.

The council had made arrangements for a widow in her early sixties to have a flat in the same block as her daughter. 'They put me here so she could see I was all right. I practically live in there. It's only the children get on my nerves sometimes and I come in here and shut the door.'

Another woman has three sons and two daughters living near to her. Her oldest son lives next door and calls in every night on his way home from work, and she also sees a daughter every day.

A chair-ridden man of about 50, has a brother and a nephew who come in the morning, get him up, give him breakfast and bring in the coal and his sister-in-law brings in his dinner.

A further 37% of patients living on their own had relatives whom they saw at least once a week. Sons, daughters, nieces, nephews, brothers, sisters, were all mentioned. Some of these contacts were regular visits.

'My son comes up once a week, or a grandson pays a visit. They live down the town.'

149

Others had more frequent contacts. A widow in her late sixties looks after her daughter's children on five days a week, while the daughter goes to work.

But the remaining 38% only saw relatives infrequently, if at all. Twelve per cent saw relatives at least once a month, 14% less frequently than that, while 12% did not have any or else never saw them.

A widower in his seventies only has a cousin in Chester, who has never been to see him.

A widow, also in her seventies, has a sister in Canada, but no other relatives.

Another man said, 'I live too far away to see my relatives, and since the wife died my place isn't fit to take anyone to.'

When people living alone are looked at in three age groups—under 65, 65–74 and 75 or more—it becomes clear that those in the middle group are most likely to have fairly frequent contact with relatives. Five-sixths of them saw some relative at least once a week, but this proportion was only a half in the other two groups. The probable reason for the less frequent contact with relatives among those under 65 is that more of them were single, just over half compared with a fifth of other groups, so they have no children or in-laws. Decreasing contact with relatives as people of 65 or more get older is likely to be a function of their own, and their relatives', increasing immobility and of the contracting number of relatives of their own age.

Thus, although a majority of those people who lived alone had some contact with relatives at least once a week, half of those aged 75 or more did not see any relative as frequently as that. For their social contacts, and for help when they are taken ill or are convalescent, they had to rely on friends, neighbours and official sources.

Summary and conclusions

Although nearly nine-tenths of the patients could have visitors every day, a third were somewhat critical of the visiting arrangements. The most frequent criticisms were that they were too short or at inconvenient times. More liberal visiting times would add to the satisfaction and contentment of many patients, and greater flexibility would enable their relatives and friends to visit when it was most convenient for them. Short visiting times for a fixed period each day can be a strain and tie for relatives, especially if they live some distance from the hospital. Even so, most patients had visitors every visiting time.

When the patient is a housewife relatives not only provide support and comfort by visiting her; often they also have to make arrangements for the cooking, shopping, and care of the children. Many families in which the patient was the housewife were helped by other relatives living nearby and sometimes relatives from farther away came and stayed with them. Relatives are a far more common source of help than official agencies. But patients who are most likely to need help are not always the people who have helpful relatives near at hand. This is particularly true of people living on their own,[1] and there is also some evidence to suggest that housewives with young families may be relatively isolated from relatives other than those in their own household. Although people living on their own were rather more likely than others to have had a home help, they were still the ones who most often had no help at all, and to feel the need for it. Far from the welfare services sapping initiative and reducing people's sense of responsibility, as is sometimes suggested,[2] they merely provide a very small part of the help that is given to hospital patients and their families. Welfare services may partially fill the gap when people do not have relatives to help, but they certainly do not replace or compete with relatives as the main source of help.

[1] See Geffen, D. H., and Warren, M. D., 'The Care of the Aged'.

[2] For instance, Dr. C. P. Wallace, in a presidential address to the Surrey Branch of the B.M.A. on 13th June 1962, said: 'Much of our welfare legislation, the N.H.S. in particular, has undermined the freedom and sense of responsibility of the individual citizen. The N.H.S. has also encouraged an attitude of getting as much as possible from the State; we have become a nation of citizens at the receiving end. This explains in no small measure the enormous and increasing cost of the service.'

XII

WORK AND WAGES

THE last chapter showed how patients' families and friends were affected by their absence from home and by the need to look after them when they returned. These problems were naturally greatest if the patient was a housewife and mother, when other arrangements had to be made for the care of children and other household tasks. This chapter considers how families are affected financially when a member is ill and has to go into hospital. Clearly the families which are likely to be hardest hit are those in which the patient is the chief breadwinner. Altogether 28% of the patients were under 65 and the main wage or salary earner in the family.[1]

When the head of household is off sick

The majority of these patients, 92%, were men; most of them, 86%, had one or more dependants,[2] and nearly all, 96%, normally worked full time. In just over half, 52%, of these families the patient was the only wage or salary earner; in the others the patient's wife or a child, or both, were working as well. Eight per cent lived on their own.

For 44% of these patients, absence from work meant cutting off their normal income completely, 36% continued to receive full pay, and 20% received something from their employers, but less than their normal wage.[3] Full pay usually meant the basic rate less the amount payable to the man from the National Insurance Scheme, this amount either being deducted from the wages paid or returned to the firm later by the employee. Even these people may, in fact, receive

[1] Men over 65 and women over 60 have not been included, as they normally receive retirement pensions. People under this age living on their own have been included, as they are the head of their 'household'.

[2] Dependants include a wife whether working or not, children under 15, and older children not yet working.

[3] Question 90: 'While you were/are off work, did/do you get any wages?' Yes full/Yes part/No. Those who received full pay for part of the time and then some or no pay after that have been classified as receiving part of their wages.

less than usual while they are sick, as payments for overtime and piecework are not normally included.

Examples of the sorts of benefits received are given below.

A park patrolman, employed by a city corporation for five to ten years, received full wages for nine weeks, then nothing.

A miner aged between 35 and 44 received half-pay for six weeks, quarter pay for a further six weeks, and then nothing. He had worked at the same pit for 10 to 15 years.

A clerical worker, aged between 55 and 59, received full pay for six months. He had been in the same job between five and ten years.

An employee of British Railways received £2 a week for a maximum of 12 weeks illness in one year. He had worked on the railways for 40 years.

Although people who had been away from work for longer than three months were no less likely to get some money from their employer, they more frequently received part of their wages rather than full pay. Those who had been in their jobs for less than a year did not appear to qualify, in their employers' eyes, for payment during sickness as often as those with longer periods of service, although there seemed to be no special treatment for employees who had held the same job for many years, often the greater part of their working lives. The most obvious and striking difference in the proportion receiving payment was between those in manual and non-manual occupations, which is examined in Chapter 15.

What sources of income were there for heads of households not receiving their full wages? All but four had drawn National Insurance sickness benefit.[1] For the majority, 71%, this was their only source of income, but 17% had received something from a trade union. Thirteen per cent got some help from the National Assistance Board; all of these were manual workers and all but one were away from work for more than two months. Several others knew of the possibility of getting something from the Board, but were reluctant to apply.

'We have managed by using savings—it's all gone now. I don't know if it's pride or what. I wouldn't go to the National Assistance. I only want to get back to work. I've got that little bit of pride.'

'If I can manage on 2d., I'll manage on 2d.—we're highly independent. I think National Assistance grows on you—we always have managed without it.'

[1] Of these four, two were away from work for less than a week, one woman was on half-pay and not working during school holidays, and the fourth was a woman who was separated from her husband and had a son of school age. She only paid insurance for Industrial Injuries, so was not entitled to sickness benefit. She was off work for between two and three months.

'It so happens we had a little set by. And I'm just lucky to have a wife that goes out to work when it's necessary. It doesn't bring in much, but it helps. The lady almoner advised me to go to the National Assistance. But we've got no doubts about doing right. You wouldn't go and take the money when there's others need it more.'

Other research has shown that many old people who would qualify for National Assistance do not apply.[1] The reasons given for not applying include ignorance, pride, and a desire to 'manage while we can'. It seems that, as well as old, retired people, some younger people who are off sick also feel reluctant to ask the National Assistance Board for help.[2]

Those who did not get their full wages while they were off sick were asked whether they had found it a serious strain, a moderate strain, a little strain, or no strain at all on family finances. Four-fifths said there was some strain, and two-fifths described it as serious.

The level of sickness benefit was criticized by several patients,[3] and the delay in obtaining it by others.

'Sickness benefit two weeks after. You would think they were giving you £10 a week the things they want to know. They sent me three letters, then paid me all at once the amount due. When they think you are well enough they write and say why aren't you back at work, and then they get in touch with your doctor and ask him. He has to put them in touch with the hospital. I think it is terrible; it would be different if you were always off sick.'

As might be expected, the strain was greater the longer the time spent away from work. The proportion saying it was a serious financial strain increased from 17% among those away less than a month to 61% among those away for more than six months; while the proportion saying it was no strain at all decreased from 44% to 14%. In addition, the degree of strain increased with the number of dependants, so that two-thirds of those with three or more dependants regarded the strain as serious. Less predictably, those in households with another wage earner were no less likely to feel their finances had

---

[1] Cole, D., with Utting, J., *The Economic Circumstances of Old People*, pp. 94–5; and Townsend, P., *The Family Life of Old People*, pp. 161–5.

[2] See also Willmott, P. and P., 'Off Work through Illness'.

[3] A survey carried out by PEP of families with dependent children in Greater London showed that the major complaint of families who had obtained sickness benefit was of the small amount received. Seven per cent said the delay in receiving benefit was worrying or inconvenient. Eleven per cent said they did not receive as much as they expected. Thirty-seven per cent said the amount they received was not much help. PEP, *Family Needs and the Social Services*. The rates have increased absolutely since the PEP inquiry was carried out, from £2 for a single adult in 1957, to £2 10s. in February 1958, to £2 17s. 6d. in April 1961 and to £3 7s. 6d. in March 1963.

been strained than were those who were the only wage earners in their family. Although patients with children who were working and still living at home were able to turn to them for help, this did not necessarily mean that they experienced no financial strain.

'With having all the boys working, that helped a lot. I didn't think I would be in long, so I wasn't worried about the money until I came out and couldn't get a job like. I could have seen the almoner, but I thought there wasn't no need. You can't expect help with the job and there are too many off work as it is.' (Serious strain.)

The receipt of money from a union did not affect the proportion feeling financial strain. Those receiving National Assistance, on the other hand, unanimously said it was a serious strain. This can be taken as an indication of people's reluctance to seek National Assistance until their situation becomes rather desperate; and it also shows that the receipt of this assistance does little to resolve feelings of financial strain.[1] What mattered most was whether they received any help from their employer. Those getting full pay were not asked about this, but less of those who received something short of normal earnings said it was a serious strain than of those whose wages stopped altogether.

How did they manage? Once again people turned to relatives, friends and workmates for help.

'We borrowed from my wife's father and a friend. You get to know who your friends are. The mortgage on the house is paid, but the rates are still to pay. The wife started work four days a week and pays a friend to look after the boy of three.'

'It was a serious strain—we went up to my wife's mother's house for six weeks, gave Mum what we could and kept the rent and rates straight at home—it saved on electricity.'

'How did we manage? Charity! They had a collection at work.'

Savings were used, hire-purchase payments were left, and wives went out to work.

'It was just before Christmas—all the bills come at the same time. We were six months married then. Fortunately we had some money over from getting married; we're saving up to buy a house. We're starting from scratch more or less again.'

---

[1] The PEP report on 734 families in Greater London showed that 12% of the sample had received National Assistance between 1948 and 1957. Forty-five per cent of them said that the amount they received was not much help. PEP, op. cit. These rates have increased absolutely, being £1. 16s. for a single man in 1957, £2 9s. 6d. in April 1961, £2 11s. 6d. in September 1962 and £3 3s. 6d. in September 1963.

'The hire purchase had to go—I wrote and told them and they let me postpone paying.'

'We got by. My wife went out to work. You can't live on the benefit. There's a lot of folk goes back too soon on account of that.'

And several families had to cut their standard of living, or get in debt or behind with the rent.

'We *had* to manage—letting go on insurances, no replacing clothes or furniture. We just had to live plain.'

'Lambeth Council are good. The rent's 30s. a week. If a man's out of work and shows a labour card stamped he pays £1 and 5s. extra a week when he goes back.'

These hardships came at a time when people often had extra expenses for medicines.

'We had money put by, but it doesn't last for ever. I have to pay 6s. a week for medicines and pills, etc. This reduces our income by 6s. a week and it's small enough nowadays on sickness benefit.'

At present people receiving National Assistance can reclaim their prescription charges.[1] To extend this scheme to those dependent on sickness benefit and to old-age pensioners might relieve most cases of hardship, but would be difficult to operate. There appears to be a strong case for abolishing the charge altogether. A number of the general practitioners interviewed described the hardships and difficulties arising from this charge, although they were not asked about this directly.

'The charge for prescriptions should be abolished. It prevents many people getting what they should. I've come across a number of cases where I know they haven't got what was on the prescription. I don't think it was really abused when there was no charge.'

'The two-shilling prescription charge is appalling. We have a voluntary system—the chemist does the dispensing—we collect the prescription and the money. I've got to collect it and I know some families—if I collect 6s. it's one of their dinners gone. I'm out of pocket about £1 some days'.

The charge may inhibit general practitioners from prescribing on occasions and it may also discourage people from consulting their

[1] People not receiving an allowance from the National Assistance Board, but who, after paying the charge, would be left without enough money for their needs as assessed by the Board, can also have National Health Service charges refunded to them by the Board. But the proportion of prescriptions 'paid' for in this way is small. In 1961 12% of prescription payments were refunded by the N.A.B.—11% to people receiving N.A.B. allowances and 1% to others.

doctor. One survey[1] showed that 9% of adults felt the charge had prevented them from going to their doctor on occasions when they wanted to, and 58% of all those interviewed thought the charge was unfair.

Up to now this discussion has been confined to those patients most likely to encounter financial difficulties through illness—heads of households who are normally working. The financial problems of other patients who normally work are described next.

Other patients who normally work

Married housewives accounted for two-thirds of the other patients who normally worked, a tenth were of pensionable age and most of the others were under 35 and still living with their parents. Only a tenth of all this group felt the financial strain had been severe, compared with a quarter of the heads of households. One single man receiving half-pay from his firm, and living with his mother and a brother and two sisters who worked, had not even applied for his sickness benefit.

'I didn't need it. The way I looked at it, I was getting treatment [for haemorrhoids] that cost well over £100 and I didn't feel entitled to apply.'

Those who did report some financial strain often referred to their dependence on relatives.

'I have my father, you know. He couldn't afford to keep us, but he helped. If I'd been on my own, I'd have felt it.' (Moderate financial strain.)

'Mum had to keep me for nothing for 19 weeks. I tried to get National Assistance, but I couldn't because Dad was working. I only got £2 sick pay—that only kept me in pocket money.' (Serious financial strain.)

Just over half of the housewives worked full time; less than a tenth of these—and only 3% of those working part time—felt that their illness had led to a severe financial strain. In a few instances the family was dependent on the housewife's wages, as her husband was not working because of illness, unemployment or strikes. For other families the housewife's wages may have been used for extra expenses, but nevertheless were sorely missed.

'My husband was working, so I knew we could manage. I was only worried because Christmas was coming up. I think I went back to work too soon because of that.'

[1] Medical Services Review Committee, *A Review of the Medical Services in Great Britain.*

157

The Hospital and the Outside World

Work and health

Patients who normally work may have other difficulties, besides financial ones, associated with their employment. Their job may be unsuitable for them or no longer available after their illness. A third of the patients normally working said in answer to a direct question that they thought their type of work contributed to their ill health.[1] Obviously people who had had an accident while at work were generally included, and they formed 18% of the total number blaming their job. But even when all those suffering from accidents were excluded, the proportion remained as high as 30%. Almost all types of disease figured, but there was an excess of mental and personality disorders, varicose veins and piles among those attributing their ill health, at least partly, to their type of job.

Some blamed the physical conditions under which they had been working.

A brass moulder, aged between 55 and 59, with gallstones, said: 'Breathing gas fumes, fumes of coke and metals helped to bring it on. There's a lot of muck flying about.'

A married woman, in the 45–54 age group, who had been working in a laundry and was in hospital with acute asthma, blamed: 'The fine fluff and the heat of the tumblers. When you open the front of the tumbler, which you do at least three times a day, you get a cloud of dust in your face.'

Others described long or irregular hours of work.

'If you work from seven o'clock in the morning to seven at night for two months full pelt and flat out on piecework and on Saturday mornings, it's no wonder it happened. I don't try now; I use a bit more judgement and ease up. Let's say I am a little older and a little wiser.' (A press operator, aged 28, who was admitted for a collapsed lung.)

'I did anything up to 70 hours a week. It's a busman's complaint, irregular hours, irregular meals, and sitting in one position all the time.' (Duodenal ulcer.)

Some referred to the heavy physical work they did.

'There was a lot of heavy lifting, big construction work, the M1 and a dam. I didn't know I had it.' (Hernia.)

'I was working in water, our pit was very steep, too much climbing and sliding. At the week-ends you might walk four miles, as there's no one to give you a lift—there's a lot of inclines and it's hard going.' (Nervous debility, lost use of legs.)

[1] Question 88: 'Do you think your type of work contributed to your ill health in any way?' IF YES, 'How?'

And some to the responsibilities and emotional strain.

'While you're a rent collector you see the 95% or 98% of people who are happy. You see the great majority of the pleasant side of life. Now I'm a deputy housing manager, if there's an awkward tenant I have to deal with him—and answer questions from the newspaper and councillors. Fortunately, I've been endowed with a certain amount of brain. Eviction—that's not an easy thing to decide; with the best will in the world it's sapping you all the time.' (Hypochlorhydria.)

Once again there was a distinct difference between men in different occupational groups. The proportion putting some blame on their work increased from 27% of non-manual workers to 58% of unskilled manual workers. This proportion also varied with the length of time the person had been in the job, being highest at the two extremes—among those who had been in a job for less than six months or for 15 years or longer. Some of the former were clearly people who had found it difficult to get a job which they thought was suitable. One man in his late fifties who had been in hospital with heart failure and chronic bronchitis described his job as a 'sweeper-up' in a factory:

'It makes me worse, the dust and doing the toilets. No one will give me a job, because I am War Disabled and have heart failure. The Labour Exchange sent me for a job dragging bags of sawdust. I keep losing jobs because I keep having to go off sick.'

That people who have been in the same job for 15 years or more often blamed their work cannot be explained merely by increasing age. The proportion of men blaming their jobs remains fairly constant at all ages, about one-third, except for the group aged between 45 and 54, where 61% did so. One possible explanation is that the effects of such things as dust and prolonged physical and mental strain may be cumulative. It is also possible that some people may need to find a reason or scapegoat for their illness and it may be easier to blame their job if a man has held the same one for many years.

In addition, more of the men who had been away from work longest said their job had contributed to their illness; 59% of those away three months or more said this, compared with 31% of those away less than three months. This suggests that illnesses from which recovery is slow and lengthy, and which foster intensified anxieties, are attributed more often to the type of work. Another possible explanation is that some people may have remained off work after they became fairly fit because they were looking for more suitable work which may have taken some time to find. Those who felt their job had nothing to do with their ill health—and went straight back to the same one—would not experience any such delay.

Family responsibilities may well influence a person's job mobility, even when his health is in question. The heads of households, both male and female, who held full-time jobs more frequently blamed their job than did other full-time workers,[1] that is, housewives and those without family responsibilities—38% against 26%. It is only possible to speculate how much of the illness which sent these heads of households into hospital could have been prevented or postponed if they had felt able to change their work before they went off sick. Other studies[2] suggest it may be about a tenth.

Returning to work

By the time they were interviewed over three-quarters of the employed people were back at work. The majority of these, 83%, had returned to the same job as before their illness, 13% had taken a different kind of job, half with the same employer and half with another, and 4% had changed their employer but were doing the same sort of work as before.[3] The proportion changing their type of work was significantly higher, 30% compared with 11%, among those who felt their previous job had played a part in their illness. Even so it was still only a minority who did so. More than half of the people who blamed their job at least partly for their ill health had, in fact, returned to the same job, and another quarter were still off work. Altogether 12% of patients back at work regarded their present job as unsuitable as far as their health was concerned. This may be compared with the 9% of men found by Curran and Ferguson[4] to be back at work three months after leaving hospital and in jobs 'that could only be viewed as unsuitable having regard to the condition of the man and the demands of the job'. Difficulty in

[1] As might be expected, full-time workers were more likely to feel their work had contributed to their ill health than those working part time, 34% against 12%.

[2] A study of male hospital medical patients in Scotland attempted to assess the proportion of cases where there was a 'preventable' factor in the illness. The clinicians in charge of the patients estimated that there was a preventable factor in 14% of the cases and the authors added another 20%, mainly on social and environmental grounds. Of all the preventable factors which contributed to breakdown in health, unsuitable work was the most prominent; it was estimated to account for about one-third of all the cases in which there was a preventable factor. Curran, A. P., and Ferguson, T. in *Further Studies in Hospital and Community*.

[3] See Question 89.

[4] Curran, A. P., and Ferguson, T., op. cit. In a similar study in 1954 Ferguson and MacPhail found that 21·5% of men back at work three months after leaving hospital were in unsuitable jobs. Ferguson, T., and MacPhail, A. N., *Hospital and Community*.

obtaining another job was doubtless the reason for returning to a job they felt was unsuitable. For example, a building worker who had returned to the job he blamed for his hernia said, 'The doctor said it would be advisable if I turned to something else, but of course you can't just turn to something else like that. I might later on. I'm doing a building construction course by correspondence.'

And some others who had, in fact, changed their jobs had still been unable to find a suitable one.

A building labourer, who thought his job had been responsible for his illness, said, 'It's heavy, and the dust. Now I took a job the other day and it was very heavy, pulling down ceilings and walls. They told me at the Labour they'd put me down for lighter work.' He was off work again at the time of the interview. 'When I went back to the Labour they told me I wasn't to do jobs like that. But if you wait on the Labour you have to wait eight or nine years, so you have to go out and find them. I can always get a job in the building, but I don't want the building.'

But most of those who had taken a different job, after being in one which they felt had contributed to their illness, regarded their present job as more suitable for their health.

A man who had suffered from blood pressure changed his job after leaving hospital. 'I can't say welding was responsible, but I gave up welding after I came out of hospital because the doctor said, "Get a lighter job." ' His present job is more suitable for health, but he now earns less. 'I'm now a security officer with a firm of bookies. I think I'm a glorified porter.'

Although the majority who had changed jobs had improved their condition in terms of their health, the picture was not so bright financially. Almost half were now earning less than before, and this was after the financial strain of a period of illness. Very few of those who had changed their job had received any money from their employers while they were off sick, and only two had received full pay.

People still off work

Many of the 80 people who were still away from work illustrated vividly the difficulties of resettlement. They were generally in the older age-groups, had been in hospital for longer periods than the others, and four-fifths had already been away from work for more than three months when they were interviewed. (Only a quarter of those back at work had been away this long.) Just over half were still hoping to return to the same job, compared with 83% of those back at work who had, in fact, returned to the same one. A further 10% were hoping to find a similar job, 17% a different type of work, 6%

were retiring or giving up work, and the remaining 13% were uncertain about the future.

Labourers who had been advised to find lighter work often expected difficulties in doing so.

'The doctor said it would be best to get a job in the fresh air. I'm hoping to get a job as a storeman. I should imagine there'll be a lot of clerical work. I am working on it now to practise, as I'm not much good at it.' (General labourer, in hospital for an operation on his nose, and a' bad chest'.)

Local unemployment added to their problems.

'I'd like to go back to the factory, not the same job; it's not suitable because it involves dust and heat.' (Will there be any difficulty?) 'I'm afraid so, yes—because of my illness and also the firm made 300 redundant recently.' (Plastic moulder, in hospital with tuberculosis.)

'I'll have to do lighter work, yes. They would take me back on the surface, but they've amalgamated two or three pits and I don't know whether there'll be anything. But when I start work I'll be getting less than I'm getting now.' (A coal-face miner for 32 years who had been injured in a pit accident.)

If they succeed in finding a suitable job, some of their problems may be solved, but if they follow the pattern of the others who had changed their jobs, they may well earn less than they did before their illness. It seems likely, too, that a number of these people will never be able to return to work for long and will have to manage on sickness or unemployment benefit or National Assistance until retiring age.

The almoner and the welfare services

In this chapter and the previous one a number of social and financial difficulties experienced by patients and their families have been described. Various services, both statutory and voluntary, exist to help people with these problems. How successful are they?

Most hospitals[1] have an almoner, part of those job is to provide an advisory service and make arrangements for patients to use the available health and welfare services.[2]

When patients were asked whether they saw the almoner at all while they were in hospital, 19% of them said they had done so, but some of their comments suggest that they may have mistaken other

[1] Two-thirds of the patients were in hospitals at which an almoner was based, but in theory at least 'almoner services are generally made available to other hospitals in the group'. *Hospitals' Year Book 1961*, op. cit.
[2] See 'Medical Social Work', a statement on the organization and function of an Almoner's Department prepared by the Council of the Institute of Almoners.

people for the almoner, and it is clear that they did not always distinguish between trained almoners and assistants or clerks working in the almoner's department.[1] A fifth of those who had seen the almoner had very little to do with her—if indeed it was the almoner they had seen. She had helped a fifth to deal with applications for sickness benefit, pensions, national assistance, or voluntary H.S.A. or 'penny in the pound' benefits. Other services she had helped people to make use of were home helps, convalescent homes, ambulances, birth-control clinics, hearing-aid services, and she had arranged for one or two people to be put on housing lists. In a few instances she made personal arrangements, such as for one patient who was a music teacher—'I had three pupils taking music exams and I had to get someone else to take them over. The almoner arranged everything by telephone; she would have taken any amount of trouble.' For a quarter of those who saw the almoner, it is difficult to tell how much help she did give them; she talked to them, but in some instances she just checked that they did not need any help, while in others she may have been doing 'casework', helping patients 'to recognize and overcome personal and environmental problems'.[2] It is possible that other patients who just told us about the practical assistance she gave them were also being helped in this way. Thus, from our rather limited information it is only possible to conclude that about a tenth of all patients received some guidance about the available services from the almoner, and probably less than 5% were given more professional help.

Patients are usually seen by the almoner because they are referred to her by the hospital medical staff or the ward sister, but in some hospitals a person from the almoner's department will see all the patients to find out who needs their help. How do these arrangements work in practice?

Older patients, those living on their own and those who had been in hospital for a month or more, had more often seen the almoner than other patients. The proportions were 18% of those under 65 and 26% of those 65 and over; 37% of those living on their own, 18% of others; and 11% of those in hospital less than a week, 18% of those in more than a week and less than a month, and 32% of those in more than a month. But in some other ways she did not seem particularly likely to be in touch with patients with difficulties. For example, among the housewives the proportion who saw the almoner was similar amongst those who had some help from

[1] Question 83: 'Did you see the almoner at all while you were in hospital?' IF YES, 'What did you see her about?' 'Was she able to help you in any way? How?' IF NO, 'Would you have liked to ask her about anything?'

[2] 'Medical Social Work', op. cit.

relatives or neighbours when they got home and amongst those who did not, and amongst the latter it was similar for those who felt they could have done with some help and for those who said they did not need any. Again, for heads of households, the proportion who saw the almoner did not vary much between those whose absence from work caused them moderate or severe financial strain, those who felt the strain was little or none, and those receiving full wages while they were off sick. However, very few patients, 3% in all, said they would have liked to have seen the almoner, but had not done so. Most of those with financial or work problems did not feel that either the almoner, the hospital doctors, the nursing staff or their own general practitioner could help with their problems.[1]

Obviously, it is not possible from this inquiry alone to judge the effectiveness of the almoner service. As far as her advisory duties go, her opportunities are limited by the other services available. When patients are in financial difficulties she can ensure that they have received the benefits to which they are entitled, she can advise them how to make the best use of their restricted resources, and she may help them to overcome a reluctance about approaching the National Assistance Board for help, but she cannot raise the level of sickness benefit. Again, if the home help service is inadequate in an area,[2] all she can hope to do is see that those who need help most get it—she cannot see that all who need help have it.

The other important limitation on what the almoner can do is that, as suggested earlier, she is usually dependent on medical or nursing staff to refer patients. When patients so often find it difficult to discuss things with the doctors and the sister, it does not seem that the almoners will always be told about the patients most in need of their help.

Summary and conclusions

The most obvious conclusion to be drawn from the experience of the people in this sample is the overwhelming importance to financial well-being of payment by employers during sickness. If the patient has his sickness benefit made up to his normal wages, he is free from financial anxiety while he is ill, but if he only receives part of his wages or nothing from his employer at all—and over two-fifths of the heads of households in the sample got nothing—then both he and his family are likely to face a sharp fall in their income. National

[1] See Questions 91, 92, 93.

[2] Hughes, H. L. G. in *Peace at the last*, states that 'general practitioners and councils of social service are emphatic that practically everywhere the numbers of [home helps] employed cannot meet the situation'. Para. 59.

Insurance sickness benefit—often the only source of income—will probably be between a third and a half of normal weekly earnings. Although relatives and friends may help, wage earners resent being financially dependent on others, and they are often reluctant, too, to seek help from the National Assistance Board. In any case, the amount of help they may get from the Board is unlikely to relieve them of severe financial strain.

Apart from financial difficulties, patients who normally work may meet problems in finding suitable employment after their illness. If there is more general unemployment these difficulties will obviously be intensified, and people, particularly those with family responsibilities, may be more inclined to cling to jobs which are unsuitable for their health. Advisory services for resettlement and training appear to be inadequate; few patients had been given any help with finding suitable jobs.

Altogether this chapter and the previous one show that there are some notable gaps in our welfare services, which can be illustrated as follows:

(1) Nearly half of patients living on their own received no help when they returned home and 16% felt they needed some help.

(2) A quarter of the heads of households who normally worked felt they had experienced severe financial strain.

(3) Twelve per cent of the patients back at work regarded their present work as unsuitable for their health.

PART FIVE

Differences in Hospital Care

XIII

VARIATIONS BETWEEN HOSPITALS

I N the preceding chapters the experiences of a sample of hospital patients have been described and discussed. It is clear that their experiences differed widely, and in the next three chapters some of the possible reasons for these variations are examined. What happens to a patient and how he feels about it will depend on what sort of a person he is and what is wrong with him, as well as on the hospital. These three variables—the patient, his illness and the hospital—are not independent, as different sorts of people have different kinds of illness and go into different types of hospital. So, although this chapter is mainly about variations between hospitals, it starts by looking at the patients in the various types of hospital.

The two main differences between hospitals discussed here are their size, measured by the number of beds, and whether they were teaching hospitals or not.[1] Table 32 shows that a quarter of the

TABLE 32

VARIATIONS IN SIZE OF HOSPITAL
FOR MEDICAL, SURGICAL AND MATERNITY PATIENTS

Number of beds	Medical	Surgical	Maternity
	%	%	%
Less than 50	5	11	24
50 < 100	10	9	16
100 < 200	23	25	18
200 < 500	41	39	30
500 or more	21	16	12
Number of patients (= 100%) ..	245	332	103

[1] Patients told us the name and address of the hospital they had been in. Information about the size, type of hospital, employment of an almoner, etc., was then obtained from *The Hospitals' Year Book 1961*, op. cit.

maternity patients were in hospitals with less than 50 beds compared with 11% of surgical and 5% of medical patients.

Teaching hospitals

Teaching hospitals are, of course, relatively large. Half of them had 500 or more beds, compared with 13% of non-teaching hospitals, although the very few hospitals, 3% in all, with 1,000 or more beds were all non-teaching ones. Only 5% of maternity patients were in teaching hospitals, compared with 11% of medical and 13% of surgical patients—a difference which is not explained just by the differing size of hospitals in the two groups. Patients' length of stay was also rather different in teaching and other hospitals, particularly for medical patients. No medical patients stayed in a teaching hospital for as long as two months, whereas 17% of those in other hospitals did so. Older patients of 65 or more and those aged 35–44 were less likely than others to go into teaching hospitals, as can be seen from Table 33.

TABLE 33

PROPORTIONS OF PATIENTS OF DIFFERENT
AGES IN TEACHING HOSPITALS

(Excluding maternity patients)

Age group	Proportion of patients in each age group who were in a teaching hospital	Number of patients (= 100%)
Under 35	15%	107
35–44	6%	110
45–54	13%	127
55–64	17%	138
65 and over	7%	128

Not unexpectedly, teaching hospitals were rather better equipped than other hospitals in a number of ways. They more often had trolley phones, 39% compared with 16%, and patients were more likely to have curtains round their beds, 71% against 55%. When asked for comments about the hospital accommodation and provision for patients, those in teaching hospitals were more likely to praise both the food, 34% against 23%, and the physical surroundings, 34% against 18%. Patients in teaching hospitals were also less likely to be woken up very early (Table 34), but even so nearly half of them were awakened before six in the morning.

TABLE 34

TIME OF WAKENING IN TEACHING AND OTHER HOSPITALS
(Excluding maternity patients)

	Teaching hospital	Other hospital
	%	%
Before 5.30 a.m.	11	31
5.30 < 6 a.m.	36	26
6.0 < 6.30 a.m.	28	30
6.30 < 7.0 a.m.	9	8
7.0 a.m. or later	16	5
Number of patients (= 100%)	70	526

A three-shift nursing system was more often operated in teaching hospitals than others, 10% compared with 4%, but teaching hospitals less frequently had a part-time nursing scheme in operation, 29% against 81%. These differences presumably reflect the comparative ease with which teaching hospitals can get full-time nurses.

Not surprisingly, since the ratio of nurses to beds is much higher in teaching hospitals, patients were more likely to describe the way the nurses looked after them in enthusiastic terms, more likely to say that 'nothing was too much trouble for them', and less likely to make any criticism of the care they received. (Table 35.)

TABLE 35

PATIENT'S VIEWS OF NURSES IN TEACHING
AND OTHER HOSPITALS
(Excluding maternity patients)

View of nurses	Teaching hospital	Other hospital
	%	%
Entirely enthusiastic	66	54
Intermediate	23	25
Some criticism	11	21
Number of patients (= 100%)	72	536

There are relatively fewer coloured nurses in teaching than in other hospitals. A third of the patients in teaching hospitals had come into contact with them, compared with a half in others.[1] It might be thought that this contributed to the different level of criticism, but this was not so. In general, patients were favourably impressed by the coloured nurses—61% of those who had come into contact with them made favourable comments, 27% neutral comments such as 'I didn't mind', 'They were all right', 'As good as the rest'. Six per cent gave some praise and some criticism, and 6% made critical remarks or compared them unfavourably with other nurses. These proportions were similar in teaching hospitals and in others, and altogether comments about the nurses were similarly enthusiastic and critical among those who did and those who did not come into contact with coloured nurses.

Patients were more critical of the medical students. Three-fifths of those in teaching hospitals and a fifth of those in non-teaching ones had come across medical students, and here 15% made favourable comments, 61% neutral, 4% gave some praise and some criticism, and 20% were unfavourable.[2] Among favourable comments, the most frequent one was that the students were approachable—'You could talk to them better than the specialists because they had more time.' A feeling of embarrassment was the most common objection—'I can't say I like being gaped at, but they've got to learn. It gets embarrassing at times; they just strip you off in the middle of the ward with about eight medical students standing around, and the doctor asking them questions.' So although most patients were prepared to accept the medical students—'They have to learn, don't they?'—for a substantial minority, mostly in teaching hospitals, they are an unwelcome intrusion.

Only 3% of non-maternity patients in teaching hospitals said the nurses were their main source of information compared with 12% in other hospitals. There was no difference between them in the proportion who had found some doctors helpful about giving explanations, but patients in teaching hospitals were comparatively unlikely to obtain their information from consultants. (Among those who recalled the name or rank of the doctor 41% of those in teaching hospitals mentioned a consultant against 61% in other hospitals. Maternity patients have again been excluded from this comparison.) Similar proportions of patients in teaching and other hospitals expressed dissatisfaction with the information they obtained.

[1] Question 50: 'Were there any coloured nurses on your ward?' IF YES, 'How did you feel about that?'

[2] Question 69: 'Did you come across any medical students while you were in hospital?' IF YES, 'How did you feel about that?'

Variations between Hospitals

There was some suggestion that the relationship between patients and doctors was rather more impersonal and distant in teaching than in non-teaching hospitals. Teaching-hospital patients were less likely than the others to recall the name of 'their particular hospital doctor', 37% against 54%, although they were no less likely to feel there had been such a person. The proportion of surgical patients who saw and identified their anaesthetist was 28% in teaching hospitals and 42% in others—but this last difference might have occurred by chance.

Teaching-hospital patients were no more likely than others to feel their medical treatment was successful, or to be satisfied with it, although other studies have shown that mortality rates for certain diseases are lower in teaching than in other hospitals.[1] Various explanations for this difference have been offered. Staffing ratios[2] differ substantially in the two groups of hospitals, as has already been noted, and it has also been suggested that the distribution of patients by social class was likely to be different in the two types of hospital.[3]

There is no evidence from this inquiry that middle-class[4] patients were either more or less likely to go to a teaching hospital than working-class patients. Whether a patient goes to a teaching or non-teaching hospital seems to be largely determined by the area in which he lives. Of the 11% of patients in our sample who had been in a teaching hospital, four-fifths were in the three areas Lambeth, Birmingham and Wimbledon. Both Lambeth Vauxhall and Birmingham Sparkbrook are mainly working-class areas and most teaching hospitals are near the centres of conurbations, so that working-class people are more likely to live near them. This seems to be counterbalanced by middle-class patients in the suburbs travelling further distances to be in a teaching hospital. In Wimbledon, a more middle-class area, seven of the sixteen patients in teaching hospitals were in a local branch of a teaching hospital, the others came into London. But when both social class and the availability of a teaching

---

[1] Lee, J. A. H., Morrison, S. L., and Morris, J. N., 'Fatality from Three Common Surgical Conditions in Teaching and Non-Teaching Hospitals' and 'Case Fatality in Teaching and Non-Teaching Hospitals'.

[2] This is so for the number of surgeons and the number of anaesthetists per 1,000 surgical beds, and for the number of nurses per 100 beds. Lee, Morrison and Morris (1960), op. cit.

[3] Ibid.

[4] This has been based for men and single women on their present occupation if they were under 60 or on their main occupation if they were aged 60 or more. For married and widowed women it is based on their husband's present, last or main occupation. 'Middle class' includes those in the Registrar-General's Social Class I and II, professional and intermediate occupations, and those in Class III, non-manual. 'Working class' covers III skilled manual, and IV and V, semi-skilled and unskilled.

hospital are strongly related to area, data from such a small number of areas cannot be conclusive.

To sum up, from the patients' point of view teaching hospitals are rather better equipped and give better nursing care, but there is no indication that the staff are especially successful or skilful in communicating with patients and creating good personal relationships. Failure to excel in this respect may be partly associated with the size of hospital. In the next section it will be shown that relationships tend to be more impersonal in large hospitals than in small ones.

Size of hospital

The size of hospital was related to its type. The maternity, women's and gynaecological hospitals, attended by 9% of the patients, were comparatively small. All of them had less than 200 beds and half had under 50. The chronic and long-stay hospitals attended by 3% of the patients were also relatively small, none of them having more than 500 beds, and two-thirds less than 200. By contrast all the mental hospitals had at least 500 beds: 3% of the patients were in such hospitals.

The majority of patients, three-quarters, were in general or acute hospitals.[1] The comparisons drawn in the rest of this chapter, between hospitals of different sizes, have been confined to these general or acute hospitals, and maternity patients (whatever type of hospital they were in) and teaching hospitals have been excluded to avoid confusion.

How do the amenities available to patients vary in hospitals of different sizes? There was no consistent trend with size of hospital in the proportion with curtains round the beds, in the time patients were awakened in the morning, or in the telephone facilities for patients. Ward sizes tended to be smaller in hospitals with less than 100 beds, and everyday visiting was slightly less common in these small hospitals; only 79% of the patients in the smaller hospitals could have visitors every day, compared with 95% of patients in hospitals with at least 100 beds. Larger hospitals were naturally more likely to employ an almoner and to be approved by the General Nursing Council for complete nurse training. These differences are shown in Table 36.

There was no clear indication of an association between size of hospital and patients' views of the nurses, but patients in smaller hospitals appeared to have a closer relationship with the medical

[1] This includes those classified as mainly or partly acute in the *Hospitals' Year Book*.

174

staff. Although there was no variation in the proportion who felt they had a particular hospital doctor, the proportion who knew and remembered his name was greater in the small than in the large hospitals. In addition, surgical patients were much more likely to see and identify their anaesthetist when they were in small hospitals; two-thirds of those in hospitals with less than 100 beds had done so, half of those in hospitals with 100–500 beds, and only a quarter of those in larger ones.

TABLE 36

VARIATIONS WITH SIZE OF HOSPITAL

(Acute non-teaching hospitals only, and excluding maternity patients)

	Number of beds				
	Less than 50	*50 < 100*	*100 < 200*	*200 < 500*	*500 or more*
Average number of beds in ward	8·4	12·6	19·7	19·9	18·4
Proportion with everyday visiting	79%	79%	96%	95%	96%
Proportion employing an almoner	0%	0%	68%	92%	94%
Proportion approved for complete nurse training	0%	21%	83%	83%	100%
Number of patients (=100%)	31	29	90	184	49

Satisfaction with their medical treatment also seemed to be greater in small hospitals than large ones. Only 3% of those in hospitals with less than 100 beds expressed any doubt about their medical care, but 16% of those in hospitals with 500 or more beds did so and 12% of the intermediate group.

There was some suggestion, too, that communications might be rather better in small hospitals than in large ones, although the evidence here is inconclusive. Forty-eight per cent of the patients in hospitals with less than 100 beds described some difficulty in communication, compared with 56% of those in hospitals with 100–199 beds and 63% in hospitals with 200 or more.

175

Differences in Hospital Care

Revans[1] has shown that accident and sickness rates among staff tend to increase with the size of the hospital. In one study of student nurses who worked for alternate periods in one large and several small hospitals, he found that both the frequency with which they went sick and the severity of their sickness (measured by the average number of days per spell of sickness) was higher when they were in the large hospital. He found rather similar effects when he studied gasworks, telephone exchanges and coalmines, and suggests that any effect tending to increase the difficulty of communications tends also to depress morale. In another study of food in hospitals Platt[2] and his colleagues found that the best food and the closest attention to patients' needs were found in some of the small hospitals, mostly those with fewer than 50–60 beds. The larger the hospital the lower was the efficiency of the hospital and the quality of food when it was served.

These data and the evidence from the present inquiry suggest that as district general hospitals with 600–800 beds are developed under the Hospital Plan, replacing a large number of the existing small hospitals, relationships may become more impersonal and communication more difficult, unless positive action is taken to avoid this.

[1] Revans, R. W., 'The Hospital as a Human System'.
[2] Platt, B. S., Eddy, T. P., and Pellett, P. L. *Food in Hospitals.* p. 201.

XIV

THE PARTICULAR
PROBLEMS OF MATERNITY
PATIENTS

THE experiences of maternity patients differ from those of other
patients in a number of obvious ways. Most of them are in hospital for a natural process not a disease, and after their babies
are born they are concerned about their care as well as their own. For
these reasons it might be argued that maternity patients should have
been considered entirely separately, and not included with other
patients in the general description of hospital care in earlier chapters.
But it will be shown that in many ways their reactions to their stay in
hospital are similar to those of other women patients under 45. They
may not be suffering from a disease, but they may be in pain, in
strange surroundings away from their families and homes, so their
experiences have many similarities with those of other hospital
patients. In some ways, however, their reactions *are* rather different,
and an examination of their particular problems suggests some of the
reasons for this.

Information: desire, satisfaction and sources

Maternity patients more often than others said they wanted to
know all about their condition, including the details. The proportions
were 45% of maternity patients, 36% of surgical and 26% of medical
ones. It might be thought that this greater desire for information
among maternity patients arose from a lack of anxiety about what
they might be told. But expressed desire for information, including
details, was strongly associated with age, declining from 47% of all
patients under 35 to 16% of those aged 65 or more. Age for age, there
was no difference between maternity patients and others. Maternity
patients also more frequently reported some dissatisfaction with the

177

information they were given, but here, too, if they are compared with other women patients under 45 there is no difference between them.

Among the maternity patients, however, those having their first baby more often complained that they were not able to find out all they wanted to know than those who were in hospital for a second or later confinement—30% against 17%. The proportions with no difficulty in communication were 18% of those having their first baby and 35% of the other mothers. So attitudes to information were related to patients' ages and, as might be expected, to their previous experience.

Maternity patients had different sources of information. Only 26% of them said that a doctor was their main source of information, compared with 44% of surgical patients and 59% of medical; and the proportions saying no doctors were helpful in this respect were 34%, 21% and 16% in the three groups. Among those who did find some doctors helpful, maternity patients were less likely to mention consultants than either surgical or medical patients, and more likely to mention a house officer or clinical assistant. (See Table 37.)

TABLE 37

MAIN SOURCES OF INFORMATION
AND DOCTORS AS A SOURCE OF INFORMATION
FOR MATERNITY PATIENTS AND OTHERS

	Maternity	Surgical	Medical
Main Source:	%	%	%
Doctor	26	44	59
Sister	40	30	20
Nurse	15	12	5
Other	6	4	3
None	13	10	13
No doctor helpful	34%	21%	16%
*Doctors most helpful:**	%	%	%
Consultant ..	38	55	55
Registrar ..	9	10	15
House officer	38	28	24
Clinical assistant ..	15	7	6
Number of patients* (= 100%) ..	116	352	271

* The percentages relating to the doctor who was most helpful are based only on those who said a doctor was helpful and who stated the rank of the doctor or gave a name which could be traced.

The sister and the nurses were both relatively and absolutely more important as sources of information to maternity patients than to the others. They were more likely to be mentioned as the main source of information and less likely to be described as providing none. This can be seen from Table 38.

TABLE 38

THE SISTER AND NURSES AS SOURCES OF
INFORMATION FOR MATERNITY PATIENTS AND OTHERS

	Maternity	Surgical	Medical
Sister provided:	%	%	%
A lot of information	23	16	13
A little information	49	43	36
No information	38	41	51
Nurses provided:	%	%	%
A lot of information	4	5	1
A little information	37	29	18
No information	59	66	81
Number of patients (= 100%) ..	116	352	271

Relationship with nurses

While the maternity patients relied more on the nursing staff for information than did other patients, they were also more critical of the nurses. The proportions who were entirely enthusiastic when describing the way the nurses looked after them were 39% of maternity, 57% of surgical and 52% of medical patients; the proportions making some criticism were 40%, 22% and 16%, and those who felt there had been some occasion when a nurse was not kind were 27%, 13% and 10% in the three groups. Maternity patients described the nurses as cheerful, friendly or hard-working as often as the others, but were less likely to use such phrases as 'nothing was too much trouble'. Fourteen per cent of the mothers thought the nurses could have done more for them, compared with 8% of surgical and 6% of medical patients.

When patients' age and sex were taken into account, maternity patients remained more critical of the nurses than other women patients under 45, although women patients in general were more critical than men, and women under 45 more than older women.

179

Differences in Hospital Care

One probable reason for the relatively critical attitude of maternity patients is that the very closeness of the relationship provides more opportunities for friction and criticism. Patients having their first baby are more likely than others to be dependent on the nurses for help and advice, and they were also more critical, as can be seen from Table 39.[1]

TABLE 39

ATTITUDE TO NURSES AND WHETHER FIRST OR LATER BABY
(Maternity patients only)

	Mothers having first baby	Other maternity patients
Attitude to nurses:	%	%
Entirely enthusiastic ..	32	46
Intermediate	17	24
Some criticism	51	30
Number of patients (= 100%)	57	60

The mothers themselves often explained their criticisms by describing the care they received while they were in labour and the attitudes of the nurses to breast feeding and other problems associated with the babies. The patients' reactions to these issues are next described in turn.

Labour

Three-fifths of the mothers in the sample were left alone at some time during their labour, and those who had been left alone were generally less enthusiastic and more critical of the nurses than the other mothers. This is shown in Table 40.

Comments of the mothers when asked how they felt about being left alone showed that nearly a third felt frightened or abandoned.

'You badly need someone there to reassure you that everything is all right, but they were so short of night staff.'

'I think it was dreadful. I was terrified. I'm sure if a nurse could have been with me it would have been better. They kept telling me to try and get some sleep. They came in every now and again to see how I was,

[1] This variation was not explained by the different age composition of the two groups.

180

but every time they went out and turned off the light and shut the door. If you're left by yourself you're waiting for the pains to come.'

'I didn't like that. I had no one with me. I was getting a bit nervous. I was calling, you know, and they used to pass in and out, but take no notice.'

TABLE 40

ATTITUDE TO NURSES AND BEING LEFT ALONE DURING LABOUR

(Maternity patients only)

	Left alone	Not left alone
Attitude to nurses:	%	%
Entirely enthusiastic ..	30	53
Intermediate	20	23
Some criticisms	50	24
Number of patients (= 100%)	68	46

But over half of those who were left alone said they did not mind. Most of these had felt they could get hold of someone as soon as they wanted it.

'I didn't really feel alone—they came at once.'

'I had injections and was more dreamy than wide awake. I knew they weren't very far away.'

'You are on your own, but the nurses keep popping in and out. I think it's good for you to be on your own, because nobody can do anything for you and you've just got to bear it out.'

Some who did not mind very much felt this was because it was not their first baby.[1]

'Well, I'd had a child before and I didn't mind much. She had two more that night and with only one of them [midwife] on duty she couldn't do much. I think you should have someone with you for your first baby.'

[1] In fact, mothers having their first baby were rather more likely to be left alone than others, presumably because of the longer labour, and no more likely to complain about it. A cross-analysis showed that in spite of this relationship, both being left alone in labour and having a first baby were independently associated with a critical attitude to the nurses.

'I didn't mind so much, because it was my second. I suppose it can't be helped; there's a shortage of nurses.'

A tenth of all those who were left alone said they preferred it. Some of these seemed to have equable temperaments and easy deliveries.

'I went in at 5.30 p.m. The staff nurse was there then and my husband was there till six. He left then. From six until eight nobody came in. I happened to call the nurse at five to eight and the baby was born then. The baby delivered itself. I think I'd rather be on my own, myself.'

Others had appreciated the privacy.

'Myself personally I wanted to be on my own. I thought I would give way to my feelings more—not afraid of embarrassing other people. I definitely preferred it on my own.'

'I was a bit lonely, but I think it's quite good really. You can have a little moan on your own.'

Clearly patients' preferences on this point vary and are not always taken into account. Many of those who had someone with them all the time said they had appreciated this.

'It was very nice to have a little nurse beside you all the time. It was comforting like.'

'When the labour pains started getting pretty bad the nurse sat down and talked to me and told me what was going to happen and said how in a few weeks I'd be laughing and saying "Was he all that trouble!" That was a great help really.'

'I was surprised [not to be left alone] because they were so busy. I think it helps. They do explain and that helps a lot.'

When they were asked who had been with them mainly, 13% mentioned a doctor and the rest the sister, midwives or nurses. Several maternity patients, when they were asked to give an example of an occasion when the nurses or midwives were particularly kind, described incidents during their labour.

'When I was having the baby a sister was particularly good, very understanding. Nothing like a "You've got to put up with it" attitude.'

'I was in terrible pain during labour. The midwife was very kind and gentle; she talked to me.'

Certainly the treatment they received from the nursing staff while in labour often seemed to make a strong and lasting impression.

'When I was in labour they were very kind—a dear motherly soul put wet cold flannels on my head.'

'When I was having the baby she was very kind. I had expected her to be abrupt. But she had her arms round me, and I had my arms round her.'

'I think in maternity they're too hard, you know. "You're not the only one having a baby. There's millions having them. It's a natural function." They're bullying and bossy. It's a pity that some maternity hospitals are like that, because having a baby is such a wonderful thing for a girl. And they're so busy and hard. I always feel you're like on a conveyor belt.'

The babies

Twelve per cent of the mothers did not feel they saw enough of their babies while they were in hospital, 4% because either they or their babies were ill and 8% because of the hospital organization.[1] Some comments among the latter were:

'You don't have the baby there, only for feeding. You watch the clock go round for every four hours.'

'They only brought her to me once during the three days. I worried about that. I kept asking; I thought something was wrong with her.'

'They brought Kenneth just for 10 minutes at feed time. It was as though they'd brought you any baby to look after. He was always crying when they took him away from me, but the sister said he was a greedy baby.'

And some of those who 'saw' enough of them could not pick them up when they wanted to.

'When you're in hospital your baby is never your own. If they cried, you just had to let them cry. They were at the bottom of the bed. It depended what nurses were on. The young nurses would pick them up, but the sister wouldn't; you just had to leave them for the next feed.'

Seven per cent felt they had their babies with them too much of the time, although they were not asked about this directly.

'I think they should have been taken away at night to give you more rest. None of them were getting enough to eat and they were always awake. In the day if you went off they came in with pills to wake you up. Oh, I was a wreck by the time I came out.'

'They had little cots beside the bed and you had to look after him yourself. And in the night when you have two or three babies yelling in the ward you get a bit narked.'

---

[1] Question 42: 'Did you see enough of your baby while you were in hospital?'

As might be expected, mothers who were happy about the amount they saw their babies were less critical and more enthusiastic about the nurses than other mothers, showing once again how ward organization and layout can influence patient-nurse relationships.

A fifth of all the mothers felt they were not given enough help, after their baby was born, with breast-feeding and other problems.[1]

'They just left it all for me to do. The girls in the ward helped me. But I think the root of it was they were short staffed. Then about the fifth day the baby hadn't been to the toilet and I was worried, and I told the nurse and she just laughed, and she said she'd tell the staff nurse and she just laughed. They didn't tell me it was just natural. There was an old midwife there who just helped out and she came and explained it to me.'

'One morning sister came in and said, "You will have go get your husband to buy some Cow and Gate, because we had to feed your baby in the night." That really upset me the way she said it, sharply and like a school order. Then one nurse said, "This won't do. This is ridiculous. Your baby has only had two ounces of milk. Give him some more." They had been test weighing him.'

'One would tell you so many minutes one side and another would say something else. They just bring them and leave them. There again I had to ask the other patients.'

A number of mothers mentioned the help they got from other patients, and relationships with other patients are considered next.

Relationships with other patients

Younger patients, including maternity patients, were more likely than older ones to talk to other patients a great deal, to discuss their conditions and to find these discussions helpful. (Table 41.)

This disinclination of older people to communicate with other patients is probably merely a reflection of a general decline in sociability with age. Willmott and Young[2] found that older people were less likely to be visited by friends or neighbours. Cauter and Downham[3] noted a marked diminution in activity and intercommunication after the age of 55. It also seems that people become less sociable and more apathetic as their time in hospital increases. A quarter of those in for two months or more—and these were predominantly medical patients—said they did not talk to the other patients very much. They

---

[1] Question 41: 'During the first few days after the baby's birth do you think the midwives gave you sufficient help in regard to breast-feeding and other problems?'

[2] Willmott, P., and Young, M., op. cit., p. 107.

[3] Cauter, T., and Downham, J. S., *The Communication of Ideas*, pp. 214–16.

are likely to have been rather more ill than other patients and they are also rather older, but it is also possible that some were drifting towards the 'institutional neurosis' which Barton[1] has described.

Maternity patients do not appear particularly sociable when compared with others under 45, although more than half of them had found discussions with other patients helpful. Several of them described the ways in which other, often more experienced, mothers had helped them.

'Perhaps there were little things that were too trivial to bother a nurse with and other patients who had had more than one child would explain it to you.'

'You were allowed to walk round and talk to the ones who were in labour and the other mums used to help the ones who couldn't feed. I think the patients were more help to you than the nurses.'

'You get lots of tips about the baby from them—the kind of food they should have and the cheap clothes to make.'

TABLE 41

VARIATIONS IN DISCUSSIONS WITH OTHER PATIENTS

	Maternity patients	*Other patients*			
		Under 45	*45–54*	*55–64*	*65 and over*
Talked to other patients	%	%	%	%	%
A great deal	54	61	62	48	35
Quite a lot	35	30	28	38	32
Not very much or not at all	11	9	10	14	33
Discussed conditions	%	%	%	%	%
A lot	38	34	35	24	12
A little	44	53	39	42	40
Not at all	18	13	26	34	48
Found discussion about conditions helpful*	63%	61%	64%	65%	43%
Number of patients* (= 100%)	116	220	129	140	132

* Those who did not have any discussions were omitted when the proportions finding the discussions helpful were calculated.

[1] Barton, R., *Institutional Neurosis.*

Maternity patients were, however, rather less critical of their companions than other patients. As might be expected, they were less likely to find the illnesses of other patients worrying or depressing. When compared with other patients under 45, they less often felt that other patients were too demanding. Among the non-maternity patients, older people expressed these views less frequently than younger ones. (Table 42.)

TABLE 42

IRRITATION AND WORRY ABOUT OTHER PATIENTS

	Maternity patients	Other patients			
		Under 45	45–54	55–64	65 and over
Found illnesses of other patients worrying or depressing	15%	32%	31%	23%	18%
Thought some patients were too demanding ..	37%	57%	46%	49%	37%
Number of patients (= 100%)	116	220	129	140	132

But complaints about lack of privacy and failure to use curtains or screens were made comparatively often by maternity patients. As has been mentioned earlier, this appears to be associated with a desire of some mothers for privacy while they are breast feeding. Among the other patients these criticisms, too, were made more often by younger than by older patients. This seems to contradict the common-sense impression that the older people are the more they value privacy. The explanation may be that the standards of different generations vary. This is likely to happen because of changing standards in care. Members of an earlier generation may expect less in the way of privacy when they go into hospital than those of a later one, and may therefore be more prepared to accept the existing conditions without criticism. But it would also seem that, as people get older, they become less likely to criticize things in general, and this may partly be because they become less aware of other people—even apathetic.

The Particular Problems of Maternity Patients

TABLE 43

ATTITUDES TO PRIVACY AND THE USE OF SCREENS AND CURTAINS
(Excluding patients in single rooms)

	Maternity patients	Other patients			
		Under 45	45–54	55–64	65 and over
Not enough privacy ..	22%	16%	7%	13%	6%
Curtains/screens not used enough*	19%	12%	7%	10%	2%
Number of patients* (= 100%)	105	209	111	131	123

* Patients with neither curtains nor screens have been excluded.

Summary and conclusions

Several of the variations between the attitudes of maternity patients and others seem to be explained by the difference in their age and sex. When this is taken into account the most striking difference that emerges is the comparatively critical reaction of the maternity patients to their nursing care. One of the reasons appears to be the way they were looked after during their labour. It seems that most patients initially feel well disposed towards the hospital staff and this attitude continues and deepens unless something happens to disillusion them. But three-fifths of the maternity patients were left alone at some stage during their labour, and this proportion was 69% among mothers having their first baby. Although a few mothers prefer to be on their own, others were worried and upset by their isolation, and as a group those who were left alone were more critical of the nurses than were those who had someone with them all the time.

Maternity patients may also be less likely than others to feel grateful towards the hospital staff, since they are not ill in the same way. And they will also be affected by the way the nurses looked after their babies as well as the attention they personally received. From the nurses' point of view, the maternity patients may appear more demanding and critical than other patients. They may evoke less sympathy both because they are not ill and because their lot—with husbands, homes and babies—may seem enviable. Nurses may also regard the care of maternity patients as relatively uninteresting, with little variety, and as relatively messy. Finally, the stage in their career at which nurses do their midwifery training may influence their attitude, since nurses who have recently achieved the status and responsibility of fully trained nurses may find themselves regarded as juniors when they start working in a maternity ward.

XV

THE INFLUENCE OF
SOCIAL CLASS

THE variations in experience and attitude discussed in the last two chapters have been those found in different types of hospital, and those described by maternity patients and others. This chapter is concerned with a different sort of variable—patients' social class. The classification of social class is described in Appendix 6, which shows that a third of the patients were 'middle class' and two-thirds 'working class'. How do their experiences and attitudes vary? It is sometimes said that middle-class people receive rather better medical care than working-class. What evidence can this survey offer on this?

Hospitals and hospital treatment

There were no differences in the delays encountered by middle- and working-class patients in obtaining admission to hospital, nor in the proportions visited at home by a consultant.

Once they got into hospital, the size of ward they were in was fairly similar for the working- and middle-class patients, but those in the professional group[1] were most often in small wards, although this difference disappeared if private patients were excluded from the comparison. Other facilities—curtains and screens, telephones, visiting times, and the hours at which they were woken in the morning—also did not vary for the two broad groups, while among surgical patients the proportions who had seen the surgeon and anaesthetist were similar for both groups.

It has already been shown that whether patients were in a teaching or non-teaching hospital did not appear to be related to their social

---

[1] Each of the two main social classes has, for some analyses, been subdivided into three groups—'professional', 'intermediate' and 'skilled non-manual' in the middle class; 'skilled manual', 'semi-skilled' and 'unskilled' in the working class. See Appendix 6.

189

class. However, middle-class patients were more likely than working-class patients to go to small hospitals. The proportion in hospitals with less than 100 beds was 27% and 18% for middle- and working-class patients respectively.

The difference in the size of hospital attended by middle- and working-class patients was largely, but not entirely, a reflection of the area in which they lived. Whereas only 10% of patients in the working-class areas—Durham, Leigh, Pontypool, Birmingham, Sunderland, and Lambeth—were in hospitals with less than 100 beds 32% of patients in middle-class areas—Lewes, St. Albans, Melton, Wallasey, and Wimbledon—had been in such small hospitals.[1] Also, in the working-class areas there was a tendency for the middle-class people there to go to smaller hospitals than the working-class patients; 43% of the former had been in hospitals with less than 200 beds, compared with 31% of the latter, but there was no difference between these two groups in the middle-class areas. These variations are shown in Table 44.

TABLE 44

SIZE OF HOSPITAL WITH SOCIAL CLASS OF PATIENTS, AND IN WORKING-AND MIDDLE-CLASS DISTRICTS

(Excluding Torrington)

Size of Hospital	Working-class areas			Middle-class areas		
	Working-class patients	Middle-class patients	Total	Working-class patients	Middle-class patients	Total
	%	%	%	%	%	%
Less than 100 beds ..	9	12	10	29	35	32
100–199 beds	22	31	24	25	21	22
200 beds or more ..	69	57	66	46	44	46
Number of patients (= 100%)	266	71	360	137	112	272

This concentration of smaller hospitals in middle-class areas may arise because, before 1948, the voluntary hospitals, apart from the

[1] This difference persisted for both purely urban constituencies and for partly rural ones.

teaching hospitals, were more often in middle-class areas and more of the local authority ones in working-class districts, and the local authority hospitals tended to be larger than the voluntary, non-teaching ones.

Relationship with general practitioners

Variations between middle- and working-class areas also explain some of the differences in their relationships with general practitioners. Fourteen per cent of the middle-class patients were visited by their general practitioner while they were in hospital, but only 4% of

TABLE 45

SOME CHARACTERISTICS OF DOCTORS PRACTISING IN
WORKING-CLASS AND MIDDLE-CLASS DISTRICTS
(Excluding Torrington)

	Working-class areas	Middle-class areas
	%	%
Size of list		
Up to 2,000	21	35
2,001–2,500	30	36
Over 2,500	49	39
Proportion with further qualifications	17%	30%
Proportion with direct access to:		
X-rays involving opaque media ..	32%	39%
Physiotherapy	6%	29%
Medical School	%	%
Oxford or Cambridge	3	14
London	10	54
Scottish	22	14
English provincial, Welsh	34	10
Irish	25	6
Abroad	6	2
Proportion with hospital appointment or G.P. beds	22%	43%
Number of General practitioners (= 100%)	63	51

the working-class patients had a visit from theirs. The proportions visited in middle- and working-class areas were 11% and 4% respectively, and in the area there was still a difference between middle- and working-class patients—11% and 1% in two types of working-class areas and 16% and 7% in middle-class ones.

There was no difference between middle- and working-class patients in the proportion referred to hospital by their general practitioner, but there was some suggestion that the doctor was more likely to send middle-class patients to hospital directly and working-class patients to the out-patient department first. The proportion of direct admissions was 45% of general-practitioner referrals among middle-class patients and 35% among working-class patients. Unlike the other differences, this one was confined to middle-class areas.

It seems therefore that relationships between patients and general practitioners vary both with the patient's class and with the type of area in which he lives. Some differences may arise because general practitioners in middle-class areas seem to be more likely to have access to certain diagnostic facilities, and to have hospital appointments. They also appear to have smaller lists. These differences between the general practitioners interviewed on this inquiry and working in middle- and working-class areas are shown in Table 45.

The differences cannot be explained by variations between urban and rural districts. It does seem therefore as if middle-class people may be receiving a rather better service from their general practitioners.

Information: desire, satisfaction and sources

Except that middle-class people were more often in small hospitals, there seems to be little difference in the *care* they receive in hospital. There are some differences, however, in middle- and working-class *attitudes* to the hospital.

There were no differences between the middle- and working-class patients in the proportion who said that when they were ill they liked to know as much as possible about their illness, but the proportion who said they liked to know the details, as well as how it affected them, rose from 24% of the unskilled people to 54% of the professional. Variations in their satisfaction with the information they were given need to be interpreted with care, as they may be hidden or accentuated by differences in the information itself. If hospital staff explain things rather more often to middle-class than to working-class patients, this will obviously affect their relative satisfaction, and so, too, will any variation in the amount of information they expect to be given. In fact, the middle-class patients more often said they were not able to find out all they wanted to know than did the working-class ones, and within the working class the skilled people said this more frequently than the semi-skilled, and the semi-skilled than the unskilled. However, as Table 46 shows, when all those expressing some dissatisfaction are combined, these differences between the social classes disappear. This suggests that the working-class patients may be more diffident about expressing criticism, and also possibly less articulate about their difficulties in communication.

TABLE 46

VARIATIONS BETWEEN THE SOCIAL CLASSES IN SATISFACTION
WITH INFORMATION

Attitude to Information	Middle-class patients	Working-class patients			
		Skilled	Semi-skilled	Unskilled	All
	%	%	%	%	%
Not able to find out all they wanted to know	26	21	17	11	18
Other difficulty in communication ..	36	39	47	47	43
No difficulty in communication ..	38	40	36	42	39
Number of patients (= 100%).. ..	228	260	144	53	457

A comparison of their sources of information showed no differences in the proportion whose main source of information was a doctor or sister, nor in the ranks of the doctors mentioned, although working-class patients were less likely to give the name or rank of the doctor than middle-class ones. Working-class patients were twice as likely as middle-class to say that their main source of information was a nurse, 12% compared with 6%; and possibly rather less likely to say no one had been helpful, 9% against 14%; but there was no difference between the two groups in the proportion saying they obtained some information from the nurses. This suggests that working-class patients, while not receiving any more information from the nurses, were rather more ready to regard them as an appropriate source of information. Freidson[1] in his study of patients' views

[1] Freidson, E., op. cit., p. 211.

of medical practice found that upper-middle-class patients were less likely to consult the nurse than were lower-class patients.

It has already been shown that there was a trend with social class in the proportion who mainly asked about things rather than being told. This fell from 65% in the professional group to 40% in the unskilled, which suggests that middle-class patients may be slightly less diffident than others. This, too, agrees with Freidson's findings that lower-class patients were more passive.

Attitudes to hospital staff

There was no difference between middle- and working-class patients in the proportion who felt they had a particular hospital doctor nor in the rank of doctor they mentioned here. Neither was there any difference in their attitude towards their medical treatment; similar proportions in the two groups regarded it as 'completely successful' and similar proportions in both were 'entirely satisfied'. But when they were asked how they found out the names of the doctors, the proportions who said they knew the doctors beforehand was twice as great among the middle-class as among the working-class patients, although they were no more likely to have seen any of the doctors before in the out-patient departments. It seems probable that middle-class people may take more notice of the names of doctors, and this would explain why they were more often able to tell us their name or rank.

The middle-class patients were less enthusiastic about the nurses and more critical of them than the working-class patients. The proportions who were purely enthusiastic were 44% of the former and 56% of the latter, while those making some criticisms were 31% and 20% in the two groups respectively. The kind of praise also differed, middle-class patients more often describing the nurses as cheerful and friendly, and working-class patients saying they were hardworking or that nothing was too much trouble for them.

Middle-class patients were more critical of the coloured nurses than were the working-class patients and they were less likely to make favourable comments, 54% and 66% respectively being favourable and 9% and 4% critical. Banton[1] in a study of attitudes to immigrants found no pattern of correlation with income groups. It is possible that the less favourable comment from the middle-class patients stems from their more critical attitude towards the nursing staff rather than colour prejudice. There was no difference between the working- and middle-class patients in their attitudes to the sister and to medical students.

[1] Banton, M., *White and Coloured. The behaviour of British people towards coloured immigrants*, pp. 209–10.

The Influence of Social Class

Relationship with other patients

There were a number of differences in attitudes to other patients. Only 29% of the patients in the professional group, compared with between 53% and 61% of those in the other groups,[1] said they had talked to other patients a great deal. But professional people discussed their illnesses with their fellow patients as much as other middle-class people did.

Working-class patients more often than middle-class patients said that they had found the discussions with other patients enjoyable, and that the discussions about illness were helpful. This is shown in Table 47.

TABLE 47

SOCIAL CLASS AND ATTITUDES TO DISCUSSIONS WITH
OTHER PATIENTS

(Excluding patients who did not have any discussions)

	Middle-class patients	Working-class patients
	%	%
Found discussions		
Very enjoyable	49	68
Fairly enjoyable	42	29
Not very enjoyable	9	3
Found discussions on illness helpful ..	48%	65%
Number of patients (= 100%) ..	212	440

There was little difference between the two broad social classes in the proportion who found the illnesses of other patients distressing, but a relatively high proportion of those in the routine clerical group said this—41% against 23% of the other patients. Are these patients possibly more squeamish or genteel than others? When the proportions who said there were some patients whom they wished were not in their ward are considered, the group that stands out is the unskilled one—only 18% of them felt this compared with 30% of the others. But, although these patients seemed more tolerant of their com-

---

[1] Patients in single rooms have been excluded from this comparison.

195

panions in this respect, they were also most likely to regard other patients as too demanding. This is shown in Table 48.

TABLE 48

SOCIAL CLASS AND FEELING OTHER PATIENTS TOO DEMANDING

(Excluding patients in single rooms)

	Proportion feeling other patients were too demanding	*Number of patients* (=100%)
Middle class		
Professional	30% ⎫	20
Intermediate	39% ⎬ 40%	119
Skilled non-manual ..	43% ⎭	72
Working class		
Skilled	51% ⎫	249
Partly skilled	47% ⎬ 50%	137
Unskilled	54% ⎭	52

Differences in the level of expectation may partly account for this variation. Working-class patients may expect less in the way of care and attention, and therefore be critical of other patients who do ask for more. It is also possible that there is less feeling of competitiveness among middle-class patients, as they may feel more able to communicate their needs, and may have fewer inhibitions about doing so. This would make them less anxious that the demands of other patients would take precedence over their own needs.

Professional people were most likely to complain of lack of privacy and that screens and curtains were not used enough, while among the working-class patients the semi-skilled and unskilled made these complaints least often. This is shown in Table 49.

These differences are obviously linked with people's preference for wards of different sizes. Those in the professional group most often said they would prefer a room of their own, and the semi- and unskilled least often. (Table 50.)

Thus in general it would appear that working-class patients both appreciate the company of their fellow patients rather more and are slightly less upset by the communal life in the hospital ward than some middle-class patients.

The Influence of Social Class

TABLE 49
SOCIAL CLASS AND ATTITUDES TO PRIVACY
(Excluding patients in single rooms)

	Proportion feeling they did not have enough privacy	Proportion saying curtains or screens were not used enough*	Number of patients (= 100%)
Middle class			
Professional	25%	26%	20
Intermediate	12%	6%	120
Skilled non-manual ..	20%	11%	74
Working class			
Skilled	15%	13%	248
Partly skilled	8%	7%	137
Unskilled	8%	6%	52

* Those with neither screens nor curtains have been excluded here.

TABLE 50
SOCIAL CLASS AND PREFERENCE FOR WARDS OF DIFFERENT SIZES

	Middle-class patients			Working-class patients		
	Professional	Intermediate	Skilled non-manual	Skilled manual	Partly skilled	Unskilled
	%	%	%	%	%	%
In ward with others and liked that size best ..	58	73	73	69	83	82
In single ward and liked that best ..	14	3	3	2	1	—
In ward with others and would prefer single ward	14	9	8	6	2	4
In ward with others and would prefer smaller ward	14	12	15	17	10	12
Would prefer larger ward ..	—	3	1	6	4	2
Number of patients (= 100%)	22	116	73	250	139	50

197

Families and jobs

What of the social problems associated with illness and hospitalization? There was no difference between the middle- and working-class patients in the proportion of families in which a child stayed away from school or another member of the family from work in order to deal with the difficulties that arose when the housewife was in hospital. But whereas only a third of those in middle-class families who stayed away from work to look after the family lost money because of it, four-fifths of those in working-class families did so. Variations in the help received while the housewife was in hospital are shown in Table 51.

TABLE 51

SOCIAL CLASS AND HELP RECEIVED WHILE HOUSEWIFE IN HOSPITAL

(Housewives only)

	Middle-class families	Working-class families
Received help from these people not living in household:	%	%
Housewife's relatives	33	44
Husband's relatives	12	20
Friends and neighbours	16	12
Home help	2	1
Other sources	6	2
No help from outside household ..	39	29
Number of patients (= 100%) ..	106	220

The working-class families were more likely to be helped by relatives than were the middle-class, possibly because working-class families are more likely to have relatives living nearby.[1] In both classes, relatives were the most important source of help, and in both help came more than twice as often from the housewife's family as from the husband's.

Working-class families were more often able to call on relatives for help with shopping, housework and the care of children when the housewife was in hospital, but they were more likely to encounter financial difficulties when the head of the household was in hospital. Whereas 77% of middle-class heads who normally worked received full wages, only 20% of working-class heads did so, and the propor-

[1] Willmott, P., and Young, M., op. cit.

198

tions receiving no money from their employer were 12% and 55%. As a result, only 9% of the middle-class people felt they had encountered moderate or severe financial strain, compared with 52% of the working-class.

Private patients

One type of care not looked at separately so far but related to social class is that given to private patients. Twenty-four of the patients in our sample had gone into hospital as private fee-paying patients. This represents 3% of the total sample, but this may be an underestimate of the proportion in the population generally. Six of the people who were not interviewed because they were too ill, had removed or did not want to answer the questions were known to have been private patients. This suggests that the proportion of patients who go into hospital privately may be nearer 4% or 5% since, as private patients appear to be rather reluctant to be interviewed, a comparatively high proportion of them may not have replied to our initial postal inquiry.

Who are these people? Why do they choose to pay rather than use the National Health Service? What does it cost them? Do they, in fact, obtain the advantages they expect from being private patients?

They are predominantly but not entirely middle-class patients— three-quarters of them, compared with a third of other patients. The private patients included men and women, young, middle-aged and old people, and they went into hospital for a variety of conditions. There were four medical patients, six maternity and 14 surgical, which suggests that surgical patients may be more inclined than medical to seek this type of care.

When they were asked why they had gone into hospital as private patients, the most frequent answer was to avoid delays in getting into hospital—seven of the 14 surgical patients said this—or in order to get a bed at all—four out of six maternity patients. The other main reason was to ensure more privacy or individual attention. Two patients thought they would get better medical treatment, and three said it was an automatic decision because they had an insurance scheme. Altogether seven patients were insured for private medical attention and when they became ill never seriously considered the alternative to private hospital treatment. In at least one instance the choice was made because of fear or dislike of the particular hospital where they would have received National Health Service treatment.

'I thought, of course, it's a terrific amount of money for working people, but if it's the last halfpenny I have I'm not going into the Infirmary.'

The social class distribution of the private patients, together with their desire to avoid delays, largely explain the area variations in the proportion of private patients. Durham and Birmingham Sparkbrook, two working-class areas, did not have any private patients in the sample. Neither did Wallasey, a middle-class area, but one where 84% of the waiting-list admissions were seen at out-patient departments within two weeks, compared with 68% among the sample generally. Melton, Lewes, and Wimbledon, all middle-class areas, were represented by six, five and five private patients respectively, so these three areas accounted for two-thirds of the private patients. In all three areas there was a longer than average wait for out-patient appointments or admissions. When hospital beds are scarce a few patients will choose to pay for treatment in order to get it promptly. In Melton the three surgical patients gave this as their reason and the three maternity patients said this was the only way of getting into hospital for their confinement. Two were having their first baby.

Numbers are too small to say with certainty that private patients do get into hospital more quickly, but they suggest this is so. None had to wait more than two weeks for an appointment with a specialist, compared with a third of National Health patients, and seven out of nine 'cold' cases were admitted within a month, compared with 54%.

Apart from getting into hospital more quickly, what else did they get for their money? Ten patients were in single rooms and seven shared a room with one other person. None were in a ward with more than nine beds. So they were more likely than other patients to be in small wards or single rooms. But they were no more likely to be satisfied with their size of ward. Three-quarters of both private and other patients preferred the size of ward they were in, an eighth of the private patients would have liked to be in a larger ward and a similar proportion would have preferred a room of their own. When asked to comment about hospital accommodation and provision for patients, a third of both private and other patients were entirely enthusiastic and 13% of both groups were mainly critical. A few private patients compared their circumstances favourably with others.

'It was like an oasis in contrast with other hospitals. Oh, it was lovely.'

Those who were critical were vehement.

'The labour room was grim. I think it's the nearest to prison I shall get. It didn't seem frightfully clean.'

The similarity of comments from private and other patients may, of course, reflect different expectations together with better conditions rather than identical conditions.

A smaller proportion of private than other patients expressed some dissatisfaction with the information they were given, 42% compared with 62%. Three specifically said that they felt this aspect of their care was better because they paid for it.

'It was worth it. The doctor had more time for you. I felt I could talk to them. He came in and gave time to you. You don't get that normally.'

'Of course, I had a private doctor and that makes all the difference.'

'You have the feeling that if you are paying you can talk to them. I'm wondering if I could have talked to him as much in the Infirmary. I didn't see him much when I was in there before.'

This difference between private and other patients is especially striking since private patients were more middle class, and more likely to say they wanted to know as much as possible about their illness including the details. In the sample as a whole these two characteristics went with a high level of criticism about communications.

How much did the private patients pay for increased privacy, shorter delays and better communications? We were only able to find out the actual costs in 17 instances. They ranged from under £20 for the removal of a nasal polyp to over £300 for a man who spent more than six months in a T.B. sanatorium.

	Number
Under £20	1
£20 but less than £30 ..	4
£30 but less than £50 ..	2
£50 but less than £70 ..	4
£70 but less than £100	4
£100 but less than £300	1
£300 or more	1
Total	17

So about a third paid less than £30, two-thirds less than £70 and seven-eighths less than £100. Was it worth it? All but three thought so, although a number had reservations. One man put it this way, 'It was worth it from the business point of view, the convenience—I can't afford time to wait—but not as far as hospital care goes.' Again the things they stressed most often were the absence of delay or getting into hospital at all, the privacy, the ability to discuss things with the doctors, and the actual attention they received, although some mentioned more peripheral advantages.

'About a fortnight before I went into hospital I went to see the surgeon. She gave me coffee and cakes—that's very different from the National Health Service.'

Differences in Hospital Care

It is widely accepted that it is reasonable for people to be able to buy privacy if they want to. It is more doubtful whether scarce maternity beds should be available only to those who are willing and able to pay, and also questionable whether queue jumping by payment should be tolerated. It has already been suggested that if people are willing to pay to avoid delay this provides an incentive to consultants who are in private practice to maintain a waiting list for their hospital patients.

Summary and conclusions

Middle-class patients were rather more critical of the nurses, and more directly critical of the information they were given about their illness and treatment, than working-class patients. Unfortunately there is no measure of the amount of information given to patients. It is possible that middle-class patients were able to communicate with the hospital staff rather more easily than working-class patients, but that higher expectations made them more critical of the barriers they encountered. The only variation observed in the type of hospital care they received was in the size of hospital, and as middle-class patients were rather more often in small hospitals, where communications are slightly easier, this suggests that the class differences observed have been reduced by slightly different standards of care, and are generally a reflection of different attitudes and expectations rather than of the care received.

As expected, middle-class people more often than working-class went to hospital as private patients. Their reasons for doing so were to get more privacy, to avoid delay and to have a closer relationship with the doctors. The belief that private patients are more privileged in these ways seems to have some foundation. However, the proportion of private patients was so small that they had little effect on the inter-class comparisons.

Although the hospital service appears to function in a relatively egalitarian way this could arise from a tendency to treat diseases rather than people and to be unaware of patients' varying attitudes and needs.

There were greater differences between the classes in their treatment by other medical and welfare services. There is some evidence that middle-class people have a rather better general-practitioner service. This may be largely because of the areas in which they live, but more information is needed about this. The most striking class difference is in the amount of financial hardship experienced by patients who normally worked. In this respect we are indeed two nations, one receiving full wages or salary from their employers, the other reduced to the penury of national insurance sickness benefit.

XVI

IN CONCLUSION—THE
BEST HOSPITAL SERVICE
WE HAVE

In the eighteenth century hospitals were founded by laymen to meet the needs of the sick poor. But towards the end of the nineteenth century nursing standards improved and hospital care became advantageous for a wider social group.[1] This trend continued in the twentieth century. As medical care became more specialized and technical, the rich as well as the poor went into hospital.

This study has shown that there are still several legacies from the era of charity and custodial care. The failure of many hospital staff to recognize patients' needs for explanation stems partly from outworn traditions in some teaching hospitals and medical schools. Teaching and demonstration sessions are even now sometimes conducted in a way which emphasizes the clinical interest of the case at the expense of patients' feelings. Attitudes of condescension and charity are perpetuated by those consultants who regard the time they keep patients waiting as of little or no importance, by those matrons whose heralded entrance to the ward must not be sullied by the sight of untidy beds or patients eating, and even by those administrators who refer to 'deserving cases' in their circular letters to patients.

But the most disturbing bequest from earlier traditions of philanthropy is the acceptance by patients, public and the medical and nursing professions of the poor and outmoded conditions in many hospitals today. Some of the delays in admission, and difficulties in obtaining admission, which discourage general practitioners from attempting it for certain groups of patients, show the inadequacy of present facilities. More efficient use of present resources might solve some problems, but for this money and encouragement for operational research within the Health Service are needed.

[1] See Abel-Smith, B., *History of Hospitals*. (In preparation.)

203

In Conclusion—The Best Hospital Service We Have

The unhappy effects of parsimony are also evident in meagre accommodation and in understaffing as well as in the number of beds available. Very large wards, with few bathrooms and lavatories, beds close together and no accommodation for patients' outdoor clothing —the lower standards of an earlier epoch continue today because of financial and administrative expedience. But it is no longer appropriate to regard a pleasant atmosphere or the patient's privacy as extravagant luxuries.

Patient-staff relationships also suffer as a direct result of economies and failure to invest enough money and research in the hospital service. Nurses who are overworked, hurried and anxious inevitably tend to lack sympathy and understanding. Doctors often do not have enough time for discussions with patients, and large wards with little or no privacy do not encourage patients to ask for explanations. Out-of-date and inadequate facilities promote and perpetuate outmoded attitudes in both patients and staff.

A parsimonious Treasury, staff shortages and inadequate operational research are not the only problems in the present hospital service, although they exacerbate and perpetuate another major shortcoming—the failure to recognize patients' social and psychological requirements. Difficulties here are also aggravated by two associated developments—the growing complexity of the hospital service and the increasing specialization of medical science. As hospitals become more complex there is a danger that, as Titmuss[1] has put it, they 'may tend increasingly to be run in the interests of those working in and for the hospital rather than in the interests of the patients'. Restrictions on visiting, limiting it often to very short periods each day, provide one example of how patients' wishes can be sacrificed to what is felt to be the convenience of hospital staff and the smooth running of the institution.

As medicine has become more scientific it has become more specialized, and an increasing number of people are involved in the care of individual patients. The hospital becomes inevitably—and in a sense rightly—more bureaucratic: responsibilities are defined and divided and arrangements are made for the regular and continuous fulfilment of these duties. This has happened for the physical care of patients. But in many hospitals no comparable systematic arrangements have been introduced for giving patients information. One explanation for this is historical—there was no tradition of this type of care in the hospitals founded for the care of the sick poor. Another reason is that it is sometimes regarded as inappropriate to lay down rules of procedure for meeting psychological and social needs. But in such complex institutions as our hospitals today these needs

[1] Titmuss, R. M., *Essays on the Welfare State*, p. 122.

are likely to be neglected unless they are formally recognized. It is suggested in this book that responsibility here needs to be much more explicitly defined, and with this formal recognition of responsibility there should go an increase in record-keeping about what patients have been told, so that other members of the hospital staff and the general practitioner can find out what has been done. The medical profession should adapt and adopt the well-known axiom from the legal profession—the best available medical care should not only be given, but the patient and his relatives should feel that this has been given. Explanations need to be seen not as a lavish appendage, but as an integral part of medical care. Recognition and acceptance of this responsibility could stimulate interest in patients' social lives, so that hospital staff become more aware of the difficulties patients may encounter when they leave hospital. This in turn could lead to greater integration between the hospital and welfare services and between the hospital and the general practitioners.

At the moment lack of integration between these various services is the other main failing of hospital care. Continuity of care is a concept enshrined in the vocabulary of the medical profession. Its existence today is almost entirely dependent on brief letters of referral from the general practitioner to the hospital and on letters, often delayed, of discharge from the hospital to the general practitioners. Only very rarely does the general practitioner bridge the gap in communication between patients and hospital staff. To describe the general practitioner as an interpreter between his patients and the hospital is, for in-patients at least, unrealistic and may delay and inhibit hospital staff from accepting responsibility.

These criticisms need to be seen against a background of general satisfaction. On the other hand, some patients seem to accept low standards without criticism. Their tolerance arises partly from a sense of gratitude and appreciation. The hospital service is surrounded by a halo, which has been acquired through the care given by individual members of the hospital staff. It is ironic that the professional integrity of doctors and nurses who work under difficulties encourages complacency about the hospital service among both patients and public, and discourages demands for improvements and greater expenditure on the hospital service. In a National Health Service public opinion could and should be a potent weapon for incentive and improvement.[1] If it is to be effective, it must be based on a knowledge of the facts, and the public needs to recognize that the interests of both patients and staff can be served by informed criticism and demands for improvements.

[1] See Brotherston, J. H. F., 'Towards New Incentives'.

Appendices

APPENDIX 1

THE SAMPLE OF PATIENTS

Method of selection

The sample of patients for this inquiry was obtained by selecting a random[1] sample of people from the electoral register in 12 areas in England and Wales, writing to them, and asking them whether they had been in hospital in the previous six months. This method was chosen as a means of providing a representative sample of adults (aged 21 or over) in England and Wales who had been in hospital shortly before the survey was undertaken.

The areas chosen for this study were 12 constituencies selected at random from the 547 constituencies in England and Wales. It was decided to cover 12 areas because that seemed the minimum number that would give the sample any claim to be considered nationally representative, and the maximum number that it was practical to consider individually or for one person to visit personally. Constituencies were taken rather than administrative areas because they do not vary so much in size. To choose them the 547 constituencies were listed in two main groups—purely urban constituencies and those containing some rural districts. Each of these two groups was divided into eleven regions[2] and within each region the purely urban constituencies were listed in order of the proportion of jurors on the electoral register,[3] and the partly rural constituencies were listed in order of the proportion of electors living in rural districts. The sampling interval was $547/12 = 45·5$ and a number under 45 was taken from a book of random numbers to give a starting-point. The constituencies chosen were Sunderland North, Wallasey, Leigh, Birmingham Sparkbrook, Lambeth Vauxhall, Wimbledon, Pontypool, Durham, St. Albans, Torrington, Melton and Lewes. Five returned a Labour Member of Parliament at the 1959 general election and seven a Conservative. Their distribution by hospital regions is shown below:

Hospital Region	Constituencies Included
Newcastle	Durham, Sunderland North
Leeds	—
Sheffield	Melton
East Anglian	—
N.W. Metropolitan	St. Albans
N.E. Metropolitan	—
S.E. Metropolitan	Lambeth Vauxhall, Lewes
S.W. Metropolitan	Wimbledon

[1] Random is used here in the statistical sense, which means not that people were selected haphazardly, but that each person on the list had an equal chance of being included in the sample.

[2] The ten standard regions used by the Registrar-General, and the Greater London area.

[3] See Gray, P. G., Corlett, T., and Jones, P., op. cit.

209

Appendix 1

Hospital Region	Constituencies Included
Wessex	—
Oxford	—
South Western	Torrington
Wales	Pontypool
Birmingham	Birmingham Sparkbrook
Manchester	Leigh
Liverpool	Wallasey

Every twenty-second person on the electoral register in these areas was then written to and asked whether he or she had been in hospital in the previous six months. The letter and questionnaire are shown below. A stamped addressed envelope was enclosed.

Dear (The name was typed in, with christian names and initials as on the electoral register and preceded by Mr. or M/s.)

I am writing to ask for your help with a study we are making about hospitals. We would like to know whether you personally have been to hospital as an in-patient at all during the six months October 1960–March 1961.[1]

Please answer the one question on our tear off-form below and return it to us straight away. Just one tick ($\sqrt{}$) is needed. Even if you have not been to hospital during this time we would still like to know this.

Thank you for your help.

Yours sincerely,

Ann Cartwright.

PLEASE TEAR OFF

HOSPITAL INQUIRY   CONFIDENTIAL

PLEASE PUT A TICK $\sqrt{}$ BESIDE YOUR ANSWER
TO THE QUESTION

1. Have you been to hospital as an in-patient at all during the six months October 1960–March 1961?

Yes ....

No ....

PLEASE RETURN THIS FORM STRAIGHT AWAY
IN THE STAMPED ADDRESSED ENVELOPE PROVIDED

. If you have moved from the address where we wrote to you, please put your new address below:

....

....

....

THANK YOU FOR YOUR HELP

[1] This period varied from October 1960–March 1961 to December 1960–May 1961, as interviewing took place during the three months May–July 1961.

210

The Sample of Patients

After about ten days those who had not replied were sent the following reminder letter:

Dear

About a week ago I wrote to a number of people, including yourself, asking them if they had been to hospital as an in-patient during the six months October 1960–March 1961.

Most of the people have now replied, but I have not yet heard from you. It would be a great help if you would complete the form now and let me have it back.

Yours sincerely,
Ann Cartwright.

Another week after this, those who had still not replied were sent a further reminder with a questionnaire and stamped addressed envelope.

Dear

Hospital Inquiry

About two weeks ago I wrote to you asking for your help with an inquiry about hospitals. As I have not yet heard from you I expect the form never reached you or has got mislaid, so I am sending you another form with a stamped addressed envelope.

I hope you will be able to spare a moment to send it off.

Yours sincerely,
Ann Cartwright.

The response

Table A shows that 87% of the people replied, 0·8% had died, a similar proportion wrote refusing to answer the question or returned a blank questionnaire, and 2·6% could not be traced. Only 8·7% did not reply at all.

TABLE A

RESPONSE TO THE POSTAL INQUIRY

	%
Replied	
Had been in hospital	3·8
Had not been in hospital	83·2
Total	87·0
Wrote refusing to answer	0·8
Wrote not answering this question*	0·1
Subject had died	0·8
Subject moved, address unknown ⎱ Subject not known at that address or address untraced ⎰	2·6
No response	8·7
Number of people written to (= 100%)	29,400

* In a proportion of cases a further question was added on education to identify a sample for another inquiry. A few people answered one question, but not the other.

211

Appendix 1

Table B shows the proportion of replies received at different times.

TABLE B

PROPORTION OF RESPONSES RECEIVED BY VARIOUS DATES

Number of days after initial letter dispatched	Proportion of responses received on that date		Cumulative response
1–2	16.3		16·3
3	23·1	⎫51·3	39·4
4	11·9		51·3
5	5·3		56·6
6	0·4	⎬ 8·2	57·0
7	2·5		59·5
8	2·3		61·8
9	1·5		63·3
10	2·0		65·3
11	3·8	⎬16·6	69·1
12	4·2		73·3
13	0·7		74·0
14	2·1		76·1
15	1·5		77·6
16	1·1		78·7
17	1·2		79·9
18	3·4		83·3
19	2·6		85·9
20	0·5	⎬15·2	86·4
21	0·9		87·3
22	1·2		88·5
23	1·0		89·5
24	0·4		89·9
25–29	0·7		90·6
30+	0·7		91·3
No 'response'	8·7		100·0
Number of people written to (= 100%)			29,400

Over half the people responded within the first four days and 60% before they would have received the first reminder letter. About 17% responded between the first and second reminder letters and 15% after the second.

The proportion of responses relating to people who had died or who could not be traced, and the proportion of refusals and inadequate responses, tended to be greater in the later returns. Among the replies the proportion who had been in hospital did not vary significantly with the time the reply was received. It seems that those who had been in hospital

212

were neither more nor less eager to reply to the questionnaire than those who had not. These results are shown in Table C.

TABLE C

TYPE OF REPLY AND DATE RECEIVED

	Number of days after initial dispatch						All replies
	1–5	6–9	10–13	14–17	18–21	22 or more	
	%	%	%	%	%	%	%
Replied							
Had been in hospital	4·3	4·5	4·2	4·4	3·5	3·6	4·2
Had not been in hospital	92·4	90·1	91·2	89·2	88·2	83·3	91·1
Total	96·7	94·6	95·4	93·6	91·7	86·9	95·3
Subject died	0·6	1·0	1·1	1·3	1·6	1·8	0·9
Subject moved, untraced	2·3	4·1	1·9	4·2	3·5	7·0	2·8
Refusal	0·4	0·3	1·6	0·9	3·2	4·3	1·0
Number of 'responses' (= 100%)	16,617	1,965	3,155	1,740	2,195	1,155	26,827
Proportion of positive replies	4·4%	4·8%	4·4%	4·7%	3·8%	4·1%	4·4%

There is no consistent variation in the proportion replying with the date at which letters were sent out, although the electoral registers were becoming more out of date as time went on.[1]

The proportion of replies varied somewhat in the different areas. It was greatest, over 90%, in Durham and Torrington and least, less than 85%, in Wimbledon, Birmingham Sparkbrook and Lambeth Vauxhall. Analysis by type of area showed that the response was rather better in partly rural areas than in purely urban ones, in the north than in the south, in Labour than in Conservative constituencies, and in lower social class areas than in more middle-class ones. (This last factor was shown by considering the proportion of jurors on the electoral register in 1954.) These differences are, of course, all connected and are not independent.

The response rate was also affected by the addition of another question unconnected with this inquiry which was included in a random proportion of the cases in all areas. The proportion of people not replying to all was 9·3% when the additional question was included and 6·4% when it was not. Thus the additional question increased the failure rate by a third.

The response to this postal inquiry was good, although by no means exceptional. Scott[2] in his research on mail surveys reported usable response

[1] The qualifying date for the registers used was 10 October 1960 and they were in force from 16 February 1961 until 15 February 1962.
[2] Scott, C., 'Research on Mail Surveys'.

213

TABLE D
REPLY TO POSTAL INQUIRY IN DIFFERENT AREAS

	Date initial letter was dispatched												All Areas
	17.4.61		1.5.61		15.5.61		29.5.61		12.6.61		26.6.61		
	Durham	Wallasey	Leigh	Sunderland N.	Lambeth V.	St. Albans	Pontypool	Torrington	Birmingham S.	Melton	Lewes	Wimbledon	
	%	%	%	%	%	%	%	%	%	%	%	%	%
Replied .. .. :	91·2	85·9	89·0	89·7	81·6	85·5	89·0	91·3	83·1	87·0	85·5	83·9	87·0
Subject died .. :	0·7	0·7	1·1	0·5	0·8	1·0	0·7	0·5	0·6	0·7	1·1	1·1	0·8
Subject moved, untraced	1·5	1·7	1·8	2·9	5·0	3·1	3·0	1·5	3·9	2·3	2·8	2·5	2·6
Refusal, no answer .. :	0·4	0·9	0·5	0·4	1·3	1·4	0·4	0·7	0·7	1·2	1·5	1·2	0·9
No response .. .. :	6·2	10·8	7·6	6·5	11·3	9·0	6·9	6·0	11·7	8·3	9·1	11·3	8·7
Number of people written to (= 100%) .. .. :	2,756	3,228	2,594	2,514	1,951	2,428	2,138	1,959	2,096	3,214	2,664	1,858	29,400

TABLE E

RESPONSE TO POSTAL INQUIRY IN DIFFERENT TYPES OF AREA

	Urban/Rural		Region*			M.P.		Proportion of jurors on electoral register		
	Purely urban	Partly rural	North	Mid-land	South	Labour	Conser-vative	Less than 2%	2% < 9%	9% or more
	%	%	%	%	%	%	%	%	%	%
Replied	86·2	88·0	88·8	86·1	85·6	88·5	86·2	89·7	85·3	85·8
Subject died	0·8	0·8	0·7	0·8	0·9	0·8	0·8	0·8	0·6	0·9
Subject moved, untraced	2·9	2·3	2·0	3·0	2·9	2·7	2·5	2·3	3·5	2·4
Refusals, etc.	0·8	1·0	0·6	1·0	1·2	0·5	1·0	0·4	0·9	1·2
No response	9·3	7·9	7·9	9·1	9·4	7·5	9·5	6·8	9·7	9·7
Number of people written to (= 100%)	16,379	13,021	11,092	9,876	8,432	11,953	17,447	10,002	6,006	13,392

* North = Durham, Wallasey, Sunderland North, Leigh.
Midland = Birmingham Sparkbrook, Melton, Pontypool, St. Albans.
South = Lambeth Vauxhall, Wimbledon, Lewes, Torrington.

rates of between 85% and 94%, and the two studies in his series which used the electoral register as a sampling frame elicited usable responses of 85% and 89%, so the 87% obtained on this inquiry may be regarded as average for such studies. It compares favourably with the response to many interview inquiries.

The postal inquiry was, however, only the initial stage of this study; the next stage was to interview in their own homes all the people who said they had been in hospital during the relevant period. When this was done it was found that as many as 15% of this group had not, in fact, been in hospital then. Most of these had been in hospital rather earlier and in a few cases it was a husband or wife who had been in hospital. One per cent of the people had died before they were visited and a further 6% were found to be too ill or deaf or senile to co-operate. Of those who were approached and were eligible for interview 4% refused and 81% were interviewed.

TABLE F

RESPONSE TO THE INTERVIEW SURVEY

	Number	Proportion of all responses	Proportion of those eligible and approached
		%	%
Visited, found to be ineligible	168	15·0	
Dead	15	1·3	
Interviewed	739	66·1	81·3
Moved out of area	24	2·1	2·6
Refused	33	2·9	3·6
Temporarily away	31	2·8	3·4
Too ill, deaf, senile ..	63	5·6	6·9
Always out, not traced ..	14	1·3	1·5
Other failures	6	0·5	0·7
Replied too late	13	1·2	
Other names not given to interviewers	13*	1·2	
Total	1,119	1,119 = 100	910 = 100

* The names and addresses of these people were overlooked when the lists were made up for the interviewers.

The response rate to this inquiry altogether may be regarded as being of the order of 71% (87% of 81%), which is comparatively low. The failure to obtain replies from 13% of the people on the postal inquiry could be a serious source of bias, since the aim of this inquiry was to identify all the people who had been in hospital recently. Only a small proportion, 4%, said they had been in hospital during the previous six months, but theoretically the proportion could be as high as 17% if all those who did not reply had been in hospital. There are, however, three reasons for believing that the estimated hospitalization rate derived from the people who did reply is reasonably accurate.

The first is that, as has been shown in Table C, the proportion of people who said they had been in hospital did not vary with the time they took to reply.

The second is based on information obtained in one of the preliminary inquiries. A hundred and two adult patients who had been discharged from a large, mainly acute, hospital at different times during 1960 were selected at random. These people were written to and asked whether they had been in hospital during that year, and/or whether they had attended hospital as an out-patient. Reminders were sent in the same way as for the main inquiry. The response is shown in Table G.

TABLE G

RESPONSE BY SAMPLE OF HOSPITAL PATIENTS
Preliminary Inquiry

	%
Replied	
Had been in hospital last year	68
Had not been in hospital	4
Total	72
Wrote refusing to answer	1
Subject had died	4
Subject moved, address unknown }	11
Subject not known at that address or address untraced }	
No response	12
Number of patients (= 100%)	102

Only four people gave the 'wrong' answer and all of them had been in hospital during the first half of the year. Two said they had been out-patients, so it would appear that they had genuinely forgotten the date of their hospitalization rather than that they deliberately wished to mislead us. The proportion who did not reply at all is higher than for the main postal inquiry, but this may be related to the type of area; on the pilot interview and postal inquiry, which was done near this hospital, 12% of those on the electoral register did not reply to the postal inquiry. It is also possible that the relatively high proportion of non-respondents is related to the high proportion of people whose address was untraced. This too may be related to the type of area, but as it was only 5% on the pilot postal study, this suggests that addresses may be more up to date and accurate in the electoral register than in some hospital records. An alternative explanation is that people who have been in hospital recently are more likely to have moved than other people.

The third reason for believing that the sample of people who replied to the postal inquiry is relatively unbiased is that the hospitalization rates estimated from this group are similar to those obtained from the survey carried out by the Ministry of Health and General Register Office. Details of this comparison and of others which can be made with this large-scale inquiry are given below.

Comparisons with the hospital in-patient studies of the Ministry of Health and General Register Office

Each year the Ministry of Health and General Register Office collect and analyse certain information for a tenth of the patients who have been discharged from all hospitals, with certain exceptions,[1] in the National Health Service in England and Wales (or have died in such hospitals). Data are given in five broad age groups, and deaths and discharges analysed separately. This makes it possible to estimate live discharge rates for people aged 21 and over.[2]

To provide comparable estimates from the present inquiry, private patients and patients in mental hospitals have been excluded. In addition, although the present inquiry is mainly concerned only with the longest period of hospitalization any part of which fell into the defined period of study, some basic information was collected about all hospitalizations. These data are used to estimate *admission* rates,[3] excluding for this purpose all hospitalizations for which the patient was admitted before the beginning of the study period. Annual hospitalization rates from the present inquiry can then be calculated on the following assumptions:

(1) Those who did not reply to the initial postal inquiry had similar hospitalization rates to those who did reply.

(2) Among those who stated in the postal questionnaire that they had been in hospital, but who could not be interviewed because they had died, moved, were temporarily away or always out, 15% had not in fact been in hospital during the relevant period—that is a similar proportion to those who were actually seen by the interviewers.

(3) There is no seasonal variation in hospitalization rates.

When the above adjustments have been made the estimated annual live discharge rates for adults aged 21 and over is 81 per 1,000 population from

[1] These are private patients, staff patients, patients in some mental departments of general hospitals, convalescent and pre-convalescent hospitals, and designated Mental and Mental Deficiency Hospitals.

[2] The five age groups are 0–4/5–14/15–44/45–64/65 +. So four-fifths of the middle age group (15–44) have been taken together with the last two age groups.

[3] Admission rates are calculated instead of discharge rates, because dates of admission were recorded precisely, but not dates of discharge.

The Sample of Patients

the Ministry of Health and General Register Office study in 1960, and 72 per 1,000 from the present inquiry, which covered the period October 1960 to May 1961. So the estimate from the present inquiry is about 11% too low.

Sixty-nine, 9%, of the 739 patients interviewed on this study had more than one spell in hospital during the study period and altogether they had 819 spells, an average of 1·11 spells per patient. Most of the information collected relates only to the longest of these spells for each patient. How representative is this sample of patient-spells?

A comparison of the age and sex of these patients with the 1960 live discharges in the study of the Ministry of Health and General Register Office is shown in Table H.

The two distributions are not dissimilar, but this inquiry includes relatively few women under 45 and men aged 65 or more. There is no obvious reason for this apparent bias.

A comparison of the diagnostic groups found in this study and in the

TABLE H

AGE AND SEX OF PATIENTS IN THIS STUDY COMPARED WITH LIVE DISCHARGES INCLUDED IN THE 1960 STUDY OF THE MINISTRY OF HEALTH AND GENERAL REGISTER OFFICE

Age and sex group	Present inquiry	Ministry of Health and G.R.O. study
Males	%	%
21–34	6⎫ 13	⎫ 13†
35–44	7⎭	⎭
45–54	8⎫ 18	⎫ 16
55–64	10⎭	⎭
65–74	5⎫ 6	⎫ 9
75 and over	1⎭	⎭
All males	37	38
Females		
21–34	21⎫ 32	⎫ 35†
35–44	11⎭	⎭
45–54	10⎫ 19	⎫ 16
55–64	9⎭	⎭
65–74	7⎫ 12	⎫ 11
75 and over	5⎭	⎭
All females	63	62
Number of patients (= 100%)	737*	247,006

* For two people, one male and one female, age was not obtained.
† Estimated from figures for age group 15–44.

219

Appendix 1

1960 inquiry of the Ministry of Health and General Register Office is given in Table I. In this inquiry we relied on the patients' descriptions of their illness to classify their conditions. The mental-hospital patients have been excluded from this study, and deaths and people under 21 from the other inquiry.

Fewer malignant neoplasms were recorded on this inquiry than might have been expected. Some of these patients may have died before they could be interviewed and others may have been too ill to participate. In addition, some patients may not know when they have had cancer, while in other cases they may be reluctant to talk about it.

TABLE I

DIAGNOSTIC GROUPS IN THIS STUDY AND IN THE 1960 STUDY OF THE MINISTRY OF HEALTH AND GENERAL REGISTER OFFICE

Internal Classification of Diseases Code	Present inquiry		Ministry of Health and General Register Office
	No.	%	%
Respiratory tuberculosis (001–008)	5	0·7	1·2
Other infective and parasitic diseases (010–138)	7	1·0	1·1
Neoplasms—malignant (140–205) ..	7	1·0	5·7
Neoplasms—benign (210–229) ..	19	2·6 } 4·0	3·8
Neoplasms—unspecified (230–239)	10	1·4	
Asthma (241)	5	0·7	0·5
Diabetes mellitus (260)	5	0·7	1·1
Diseases of thyroid gland (250—259)	10	1·4	0·8*
Other allergic, endocrine system, metabolic and nutritional diseases (240, 242–245, 270, 289)	3	0·4	0·4*
Diseases of blood and blood-forming organs (290–299)	3	0·4	0·8
Mental, psychoneurotic and personality disorders (300–326)	19	2·6	1·2
Vascular lesions affecting C.N.S. (330–334)	6	0·8	1·3
Inflammatory and other diseases of C.N.S. and diseases of nerves, etc. (340–369)	4	0·6	1·6
Cataract (385)	13	1·8	0·9
Other diseases and conditions of eye (370–384, 386–389)	8	1·1	1·3

220

Internal Classification of Diseases Code	Present inquiry		Ministry of Health and General Register Office
	No.	%	%
Diseases of ear (390–398)	2	0·3	0·6
Varicose veins of lower extremities (460)	11	1·5	1·7
Piles, haemorrhoids (461)	6	0·8	0·9
Arteriosclerotic and degenerative heart disease, coronary thrombosis (420–422)	9	1·3	2·1
Other diseases of circulatory system, hypertension (400–416, 430–456, 462–468)	15	2·1	3·7
Pneumonia (490–493)	17	2·4	1·2
Bronchitis (500–502)	12	1·7	1·6
Hypertrophy of tonsils and adenoids with(out) tonsillectomy or adenoidectomy (510)	1	0·1	0·9
Sinus, other diseases of respiratory system (470–483, 511–527)	20	2·8	2·1
Diseases of teeth and supporting structures (530–535)	11	1·5	1·0
Peptic, including gastrojejunal ulcer (540–542)	26	3·6	2·4
Hernia (560–561)	24	3·3	3·2
Diseases of gall bladder and biliary ducts (584–586)	17	2·4	1·4
Appendicitis (550–553)	20	2·8	2·9*
Other diseases of digestive system (536–539, 543–545, 570–583) ..	15	2·1	2·8*
Symptoms and unclassifiable—digestive (784, 785)	13	1·8	1·2*
Diseases of urinary system (590–609)	15	2·1	1·7
Diseases of male genital organs (610–617)	7	1·0	1·4
Uterovaginal prolapse and malposition of uterus (631, 632)	19	2·6	1·6
Other diseases of female genital organs (620–630, 633–637)	20	2·8	4·5
Hysterectomy N.O.S.‡	9	1·2	—
Dilatation and Curettage N.O.S.‡ ..	27	3·7	—

(continued)

221

Internal Classification of Diseases Code	Present inquiry		Ministry of Health and General Register Office %
	No.	%	
Complications of pregnancy –baby not delivered (640–649)	1	0·1 ⎫	
Abortion, miscarriage (650–652) ..	18	2·5 ⎪	
Delivery (660, 670–678)	117	16·3 ⎬ 19·0	20·4
Complications of puerperium—baby not delivered (680–689)	1	0·1 ⎭	
Diseases of skin and cellular tissue (690–716)	11	1·5	1·7
Arthritis (720–725)	12	1·7	1·2*
Other diseases of bones and organs of movement (726–749)	27	3·7	3·0*
Congenital malformations (750–759)	—	—	0·4
Senility (794)	—	—	0·2
Other symptoms and ill-defined conditions (780–783, 786–795)	39	5·5	2·4
Fractures (N800–N829)	26	3·6 ⎫	
Other accidents, poisoning and violence (N830–N999)	26	3·6 ⎬ 7·2	8·5
Special admissions (Y list)	—	—	1·6
Patient didn't want to answer ..	2	0·3	—
All causes	720†	100·0	100·0

* For these categories of disease the ICD code numbers have been grouped slightly differently in the two inquiries. The code numbers given are those used in the present inquiry.

† Nineteen patients in mental hospitals have been excluded.

‡ Not otherwise specified.

Other cases of malignant disease may have been recorded just under their treatment—'hysterectomy' or 'dilatation and curettage'. These codes were only used when the nature of the underlying condition was not known. It is likely that some abortions will have been classified as 'dilatation and curettage', whereas others in this group should be included as 'other diseases of the female genital organs'. Rather more people in our sample than might have been expected have been classified as suffering from mental, psychoneurotic or personality disorders. On the other hand, when the proportion who had been in mental hospitals is considered the rate is somewhat lower than would be expected from the Registrar-

The Sample of Patients

General's Statistical Review for 1959 (Supplement on Mental Health).[1] So if both groups are considered together patients with some form of mental illness appear to be adequately represented in our sample. We have an apparent slight excess of patients with cataract, and diseases of the gall bladder, and a slight deficiency of patients with respiratory tuberculosis.

However, the differences are not large and in general it would appear that patients have described their illnesses in terms which have made it possible to classify them reasonably accurately.

It is possible to make one or two further comparisons with the Ministry of Health and General Register Office inquiry. In 1957 they found that the median length of stay in hospital was ten and a half days, and the mean stay was three weeks. In 1960, the mean length of stay was 19 days, but the median was not given. Table J shows the distribution found in this inquiry. The median is about twelve days, but our sample of hospital spells might be expected to be biased towards rather longer periods in hospital than a straight sample of all discharges, since patients with more than one period in hospital during the study period were only questioned about their longest stay.

TABLE J

LENGTH OF STAY IN HOSPITAL

	%
Less than 3 days	6
3 days < 1 week	17
1 week < 2 weeks	29
2 weeks < 3 weeks	17
3 weeks < 1 month	12
1 month < 2 months	11
2 months < 3 months	3
3 months or more	5
Number of patients (= 100%)	736*

* For three patients this was not known.

In 1960, 12·6% of the discharges and deaths in the official inquiry were from teaching hospitals. A somewhat smaller proportion, 11%, of our patients had been in teaching hospitals, but this will depend very largely on the actual areas selected. The types of hospital are shown in Table K.

[1] Figures from our inquiry give an annual admission rate of 1·5 per 1,000 population, those from the Registrar-General's Statistical Review for 1959 suggest a discharge rate of 2·9 per 1,000 population. In 1959 only 13·5% of the discharges from mental hospitals were of people who had been in for six months or more, so the difference between discharges and admissions is unlikely to account for this discrepancy.

223

Appendix 1

TABLE K

TYPE OF HOSPITAL

Type of hospital	Present inquiry	Ministry of Health and G.R.O. study 1960
Non-teaching hospitals	%	%
Acute, mainly acute, partly acute	67·0	69·5
Chronic, long stay, mainly long stay	3·6	3·5
TB, isolation and chest	2·6	2·3
Gynaecology and maternity ..	7·7	5·9
Others	8·0	6·2
Teaching hospitals		
Acute, mainly acute	9·1	9·4
Gynaecology and maternity ..	1·4	1·2
Others	0·6	2·0
Number of patients (= 100%) ..	701*	355,342†

* Nineteen patients in mental hospitals have been excluded and 19 for whom inadequate information was obtained.

† Children's acute hospitals have been excluded.

A final comparison relates to the proportion of immediate admissions—as opposed to those from waiting lists. This was 44% in our sample and 52% in the (1960) larger inquiry. (Maternity cases have been excluded in both instances.) The proportion of those who were admitted from the waiting list who had to wait six months or more was 10% in the 1958 Ministry inquiry (it has not been given in later ones) and 11% in the present study.

Summary

Twelve constituencies in England and Wales were selected for this study. Then we wrote to a random sample of people on the electoral register in these areas and asked whether they had been in hospital in the previous six months. Eighty-seven per cent replied to this inquiry.

When they were visited in their homes 15% of those who said in their reply that they had been in hospital were found not to have been in during the relevant period, although this was clearly stated both in the accompanying letter and on the questionnaire. Of those approached and found to be eligible, 4% refused, 7% were too ill to take part, and 8% had moved out of the area, were away or could not be traced; 81% were successfully interviewed.

224

The Sample of Patients

The resulting sample of 739 patients appears to be reasonably representative. Comparisons with the inquiries carried out by the Ministry of Health and General Register Office for hospitalization rates, age and sex of patients, diagnosis, length of stay and type of hospital show only small discrepancies between the present study and the much larger official inquiries.

APPENDIX 2

THE SAMPLE OF GENERAL PRACTITIONERS

THE sample of general practitioners was drawn from the same 12 areas as the patients. Only two of the constituencies selected were Local Executive Council Areas, and in these a random sample of 12 doctors was chosen from the list published for the area of medical practitioners providing services. In the other 10 areas the Local Executive Councils were approached and asked for a list of doctors with practices in the relevant districts. This they all provided and 12 doctors were chosen at random in each area.

The following letter was then sent to each of the 144 doctors who had been selected:

Dear Dr. . . . .

I am writing to ask for your help in a study we are making of the relationship between hospitals and general practitioners and between hospitals and patients. We are anxious to obtain the views of a representative sample of general practitioners on this subject. The study is financed by the Nuffield Provincial Hospitals Trust and is being carried out in a number of districts all over England and Wales. The chairman of our advisory committee is Professor Norman Morris of Charing Cross Hospital.

I shall be in . . . from . . . to . . . inclusive, and will be grateful if you can arrange to see me for about half an hour some time during that week to give me your views. Would you let me know when it would be convenient for me to call?

Yours sincerely,

Ann Cartwright, B.Sc., Ph.D.

One hundred and twenty-four of the doctors were interviewed, 86%. Eleven, 8%, were away during the study week, two were ill or in hospital themselves, and seven, 5%, refused or were too busy.

Although this sample of general practitioners was relatively complete, it has certain limitations. A number of doctors appear on the list of more than one Executive Council, and have patients in a number of different areas. Doctors on a number of lists may have had a relatively unfair chance of being included in this sample and the basis of the sample is therefore somewhat indefinite. Each doctor in a particular area had an equal chance of being included, so that doctors with small lists had the same chance as doctors with large lists. Ideally, when considering the patients' point of view, it would have been more appropriate to choose doctors with a probability proportional to the number of patients on their lists, but this information is not available. In fact, however, doctors with

227

small lists may be somewhat under-represented in this sample. A tenth of the sample were personally responsible for less than 1,500 National Health Service patients and 42% for 2,500 or more. Figures from the Annual Report of the Ministry of Health show 27% with lists of under, 1,500 and 46% with lists of 2,500 or more in October 1961. This difference may have arisen because of different definitions of list size for doctors in partnership. The Ministry of Health take the actual size of each doctor's list, whereas on this inquiry doctors were asked to estimate the number of patients they looked after.

The proportion of general practitioners in partnership and the proportion with an assistant are similar to the overall distribution in the country, as can be seen from Table L.

So, in spite of some theoretical disadvantages in the way the sample was selected, it appears to be reasonably representative.

TABLE L

TYPE OF PRACTICE

	Present inquiry	Data from Ministry of Health for 1 October 1961
	%	%
Single-handed with no assistant ..	28	25
Single-handed with assistant ..	3	3
Partnership, no assistant	58	64
Partnership with assistant ..	11	8
Size of 'firm'	%	%
One (single-handed)	31	28
Two	28	34
Three or more	41	38
Number of general practitioners (= 100%)	123*	20,107

* Inadequate information was obtained from one general practitioner.

APPENDIX 3

INTERVIEW SCHEDULES

(a) For Patients

NTRODUCTION. My name is.................
'm from the Institute of Community Studies. We
re doing a survey of hospitals from the patients'
oint of view to find out what they think of the
ospitals and the treatment they got there. This
/ill be useful to people who work in hospitals and
ɔ those who are planning new hospitals. Do you
emember we wrote to you and asked whether you
ad been in hospital in the last six months? I'd like
ɔ ask you some questions about it. We're not connected with any hospital, we just picked the names
of people to write to from the list of voters so that
we'd get a proper cross-section of people, and we're
visiting the people who said they had been in
hospital. Any information you give us will be
treated with the strictest confidence. It will not be
given to anyone else and in the book we plan to
write it will not be possible to identify any of the
people who take part or any of the hospitals or
people they mention.

1. How many times were you in hospital, as an in-patient, during the six months ....
last year, to ....,.. this year, inclusive?........
number.

Which month were you admitted to hospital? Month Year	How long were you in hospital?								Hospital		Was that under the N.H.S.? Did you pay any-thing?
	Less than 3 days	3 days < 1 week	1 week < 2 weeks	2 weeks < 3 weeks	3 weeks < 1 month	1 month < 2 months	2 months < 3 months	3 months + specify	Name	Address	All N.H.S. / Amenity Bed / Private
	1	2	3	4	5	6	7	8			9 0 1
	1	2	3	4	5	6	7	8			9 0 1
	1	2	3	4	5	6	7	8			9 0 1

2. [I'd like to ask you about the time you were in
.... hospital for
.... (period) during ....
(month).] TAKE LONGEST PERIOD.
What struck you most about your experience
in hospital then?
[Q & C]

3. What were you in hospital for?
[C]
What was the name of your condition?
Not asked......... X
What were your symptoms?
Not asked......... X
Where did they affect you?
Not asked......... X

Now I'd like to ask you what you did about
that condition before you went into hospital.

4. Did you consult your own doctor—G.P.—
about it before you went into hospital?
Yes 1
No 2
IF YES (1) Was that under the N.H.S. or
privately?
N.H.S............ 3
Private........... 4
Both 5
IF NO (2) Why not?
[Q & C]

[IF DOCTOR NOT CONSULTED GO
ON TO QUESTION 12]

5. Do you think you went to the doctor as soon
as it was necessary?
Yes 5
No 6
IF NO (6) Why didn't you go earlier?

[MATERNITY CASES GO ON TO
QUESTION 10]

229

6. How long had you been going to him with that condition?

First time 3
Less than 2 weeks 4
2 weeks < 1 month 5
1 month < 2 months 6
2 months < 3 months 7
3 months < 6 months 8
6 months < 1 year 9
1 year + (specify no. of years) ....
COMMENTS:
[Q]

7. And did he send you to hospital for that illness
—(IF NO CHECK—neither as an in-patient nor as an out-patient?)

Yes 7
No 8
IF NO (8) Do you think your doctor should have sent you to hospital?
[Q & C]

[IF G.P. DID NOT REFER GO ON TO QUESTION 12]

8. Did he arrange for you to go in straight away as an in-patient or did he send you as an out-patient first?

In-patient 8
Out-patient 9
IF IN-PATIENT (8) How long was it before you were admitted?
Same day 8
1 day < 3 days 9
3 days < 1 week 0
1 week + (specify no. of weeks) ....
IF OUT-PATIENT (9)
(i) How long was it before you were seen at out-patients?
Less than a week 8
1 week < 2 weeks 9
2 weeks < 1 month 0
1 month < 2 months 1
2 months < 3 months 2
3 months + (specify no. of months) ....
(ii) How long after you were seen at out-patients was it before you were admitted?
Less than a week 8
1 week < 2 weeks 9
2 weeks < 1 month 0
1 month < 2 months 1
2 months < 3 months 2
3 months + (specify no. of months) ....
(iii) Did you see your G.P. after you had been to out-patients and before you were admitted?
Yes 3
No 4
IF YES (3) Did you see him after you knew exactly when you would be going into hospital?
Yes 5
No 6
9. Do you think the G.P. sent you to hospital as soon as it was necessary?
Yes 8
No 9
IF NO (9) Why do you feel that?
[Q & C]

10. Who first suggested you should go to hospital —you or the doctor?
Doctor 7
Subject 8
IF SUBJECT (8) Why did you do that?
[Q & C]

11. Did the G.P./doctor arrange for a specialist from the hospital to come and see you at your home before you went into hospital?
Yes 1
No 2
IF YES (1)
(a) Did the G.P. and the specialist come and see you together?
Yes 3
No 4
(b) How did you feel about that visit?
[Q]

[ONLY ASK QUESTIONS 12–14 IF G.P. NOT CONSULTED—NO (2) AT QUESTION 4 OR G.P. DID NOT REFER–NO (8) AT QUESTION 7. OTHERWISE GO ON TO QUESTION 15]

12. How did you come to go to hospital then?
[Q & C]

13. Did you go to casualty first—or to some other department?
Casualty 5
Other (specify)
....

14. Did you go as an out-patient first or were you admitted straight away?
Out-patient first 9
Admitted straight away 8
IF OUT-PATIENT FIRST (9) How long was it after you were seen at out-patients before you were admitted?
Less than a week 8
1 week < 2 weeks 9
2 weeks < 1 month 0
1 month < 2 months 1
2 months < 3 months 2
3 months + (specify no. of months) ....

[TO ALL]

15. Had you ever been to hospital as an in-patient before?—To that particular hospital?
Yes, I.P. to that hospital 1
Yes, I.P. to other hospital 2
No, never 3
IF YES (1 or 2)
(a) When was the last, most recent time?
Within previous 12 months 4
1 year < 5 years ago 5
5 years < 10 years ago 6
10 years < 20 years ago 7
20 years or more ago 8
(b) Do you think your previous experience affected your feelings about going into hospital this time? In what way?
RECORD DETAILS AND CODE
Did not affect feelings 9
Made more confident 0
Made less confident 1

16. When you first went into hospital this time who would you say helped you most to find your way around and feel settled?
RECORD COMMENTS & CODE

Was it mainly:
The doctors 3
The sister 4
PROMPT   The nurses 5
IF   The other patients ... 6
NECESSARY   The receptionist 7
Or someone else (specify) 8
....
How did they help you?

230

17. What did you think of the hospital itself and the accommodation and provisions for the patients? [Q & C]

18. So do you think the accommodation and provision for patients could be improved in any way?

> Yes 8
> No 9

IF YES (8) How? In any other way apart from those you've already told me about? [Q & C]

19. Was there a phone you could use? (Could it be brought to your bed?)

> Trolley phone 1
> Other phone 2
> No phone 3

IF PHONE (1 or 2) Did you use it?

> Yes 4
> No 5

20. What time were you woken up in the morning?

> Before 5 a.m. 1
> 5 a.m. < 5.15 2
> 5.15 < 5.30 3
> 5.30 < 5.45 4
> 5.45 < 6 a.m. 5
> 6 a.m. < 6.15 6
> 6.15 < 6.30 7
> 6.30 < 6.45 8
> 6.45 < 7 a.m. 9
> 7 a.m. or later 0

21. Did you find that:

> Too early 6
> PROMPT Too late 7
> About right 8

22. What about visiting arrangements—how many days a week could you have visitors? RECORD NUMBER ....

23. Did you have visitors:

> Every visiting time 3
> PROMPT Most visiting times 4
> Less frequently 5

24. What did you think of the visiting hours and arrangements? [Q & C]

Now I'd like to ask you about your medical treatment while you were in hospital.

OMIT FOR MATERNITY CASES.

24. What treatment did you have? Anything else? [Q & C]

[TO ALL]
25. Did you have an operation? (Did you have a general anaesthetic?)

> Yes 1
> No 2

IF YES (1) What was it? What did they do? [Q & C]

26. In general do you feel satisfied or dissatisfied with the medical treatment you received while you were in hospital?

> Satisfied 3
> Dissatisfied 4

RECORD COMMENTS [Q]

IF DISSATISFIED (4) Why is that?

[IF NO OPERATION GO ON TO QUESTION 31 or 45]

27. Who gave you the form to sign consenting to the operation? RECORD RANK OR NAME IF DOCTOR
....

> Sister 5
> Fully trained nurse 6
> Nurse doing training 7
> Nurse—U.K. if trained 8
> Other (specify) ....
....

How did you feel about that? [Q]

28. Did you see the anaesthetist at all—either before the operation or afterwards—apart from immediately before the operation?

> Yes, before only 3
> Yes, after only 4
> Yes, both before and after 5
> No 6
> Don't know .... y

29. Did you see the surgeon who did the operation, before and after the operation?

> Yes. before only 3
> Yes. after only 4
> Yes both before and after 5
> No 6
> Don't know .... y

30. Before the operation would you say you were:

> Very anxious 1
> PROMPT A little anxious 2
> or Not at all anxious 3

IF AT ALL ANXIOUS (1 or 2)
(a) What were you mainly anxious about?

(b) Did you discuss your anxieties with any-one—either in hospital or before you went in? Who?

> No one 4
> Someone (specify) ....
....

IF NOT AT ALL ANXIOUS (3)
Why was that?

[MATERNITY CASES ASK QUES-TIONS 31–44 OTHERS GO ON TO QUESTION 45]

31. How many times did you visit the hospital before the baby was born? ....
IF NEVER VISITED
(a) Why was that?

(b) Did you go to any other ante-natal clinic during that pregnancy?

> Yes 5
> No 6

32. Did you enjoy attending the ante-natal clinic?

> RECORD Yes 7
> COMMENTS No 8

IF NO (8) Why not?

33. Were any special lectures and classes available?
Yes 9
No 0
IF YES (9) Did you attend any of these?
Yes 1
No 2
IF YES (1)
(a) How many?
(b) Did your husband also attend?
Yes 3
No 4
(c) Do you think they helped you in labour:
Very much 5
PROMPT Slightly 6
Not at all 7
COMMENTS:

IF NO (2) Why not?

34. What was your greatest fear during your last pregnancy?

35. Were you left alone at all before the baby was born?
Yes 8
No 9

36. How did you feel about that? [Q & C]

37. Who was with you mainly? [C]

38. Is there anyone else you would have liked to have been there? [C]

39. Was your husband with you at all—in the early stages—when the baby was born?
Yes—early stages only 1
Yes—when baby born 2
No 3
IF YES (1 or 2) How did you feel about that? [Q]
IF NO (3) Would you have liked him to be there?
Yes 4
No 5
IF YES (4) Wasn't it possible to arrange it? [Q]

IF NO (5) Why is that? [Q & C]

40. Looking back do you now consider your labour was:
An interesting experience 6
PROMPT Rather unpleasant but endurable 7
A nightmare 8
COMMENTS [Q]

41. During the first few days after the baby's birth do you think the midwives gave you sufficient help in regard to breast feeding and other problems?
Yes 9
No 0
IF NO (0) What more help would you have liked? [Q]

42. Did you see enough of your baby while you were in hospital?
Yes 1
No 2
IF NO (2) Why was this? [Q]

43. When you left hospital did you feel competent to look after your baby?
Yes 3
No 4
IF NO (4) What were your main worries?

44. Do you consider you have suffered mentally or physically as a result of having a baby?
Yes 5
No 6
IF YES (5)
(a) Could you tell me in what way?

(b) Do you think the hospital staff could have done more to prevent this upset?

[TO ALL]

45. Can we talk about the nurses (and midwives)—how would you describe the way they looked after you? [Q & C]

46. Was there any occasion when you felt they could have done more for you?
Yes 1
No 2
IF YES (1) What? [Q]

47. Can you give me an example of an occasion when you thought a nurse (or midwife) was particularly kind? (Is there no particular thing you remember?) [Q]

48. Was there any occasion when a nurse (or midwife) was not very kind—either to you or to any other patient?
Yes 3
No 4
IF YES (3) What happened then? [Q]

49. What about the nurses' *skill*. In general would you say the nurses were:
Very skilful and gentle 5
PROMPT Fairly skilful and gentle 6
Not very skilful and gentle 7

50. Were there any coloured nurses on your ward?
Yes 9
No 0
IF YES (9) How did you feel about that?

51. What about the ward sister—how would you describe the way she looked after you?

52. How do you think the nurses (and midwives) got on with the ward sister?

53. While you were in hospital were you able to find out all you wanted to know about your condition, your treatment and your progress?
Yes 1
No 2
IF NO (2)
(a) What else would you have liked to have been told about? Anything else?

(b) Did you ask anyone about this?
Yes 3
No 4
IF YES (3)
(i) Who? (RECORD RANK OR NAME IF DOCTOR)
....
Sister 5
Fully trained nurse 6
Nurse doing training 7
Nurse U.K. if trained 8
Other (specify) 9
....
(ii) What happened?
IF NO (4) Why not?

54. Was there anything (else) you would have liked to have had explained to you in more detail?
    Yes 5
    No 6
    IF YES (5) OBTAIN DETAILS—RECORD ABOVE IF BLANK

55. Were you able to find out about things as soon as you wanted to?
    Yes 7
    No 8
    IF NO (8) OBTAIN DETAILS—RECORD AT Q. 53 IF BLANK

56. Who did you find out most about your condition, your treatment and your progress from—while you were in hospital?
    RECORD RANK OR NAME IF DOCTOR
    ....
    Sister 5
    Fully trained nurse 6
    Nurse doing training 7
    Nurse—U.K. if trained 8
    Other (specify) 9
    ....
    IF DOCTORS NOT MENTIONED. What about the doctors—which of them was most helpful in this way? RANK OR NAME
    ....

57. What about the sister—did she give you:
    A lot of information 1
    PROMPT A little information 2
    or No information about your illness, treatment and progress. 3
    IF 1 or 2 What sort of things did she tell you about? [Q]

    IF NO INFORMATION (3) Why was that, do you think? [Q]

58. What about the nurses, did they give you
    A lot of information 1
    PROMPT A little information 2
    or No information about your illness, treatment and progress. 3
    IF 1 or 2 What sort of things did they tell you about? [Q]

    IF NO INFORMATION (3) Why was that, do you think? [Q]

59. In general did you ask about things or did people tell you of their own accord?
    Asked 6
    Told 7
    RECORD COMMENTS: [Q]

60. When you're ill do you like to know as much as possible about what is wrong with you or how do you feel?
    Like to know as much as possible 8
    Other (specify) 9
    RECORD COMMENTS: [Q]

61. Are you mainly interested in how it is going to affect you or do you like to know the actual mechanical details as well?
    Mainly how it affects me 0
    Like to know mechanical details 1
    RECORD COMMENTS: [Q]

62. Did you find it easy to think of all the things you wanted to ask while the doctors were there or did you sometimes only think of things afterwards?
    All things while doctors there ... 4
    Only thought of some things afterwards 5
    IF ONLY THOUGHT OF SOME THINGS AFTERWARDS (5)
    What sort of things? Anything else? [Q]

63. Here are three descriptions of doctors—will you read them and tell me which one most nearly describes your experience while you were in hospital.
    (1) It was easy to talk to the doctors and to ask them questions 1
    (2) The doctors were rather busy and it was not possible to talk to them as much as you liked, but when you did they were helpful 2
    (3) It was not possible to have any really helpful discussion with the doctors 3
    Is there anything you would like to add to that? [Q]

    Could you give an example of the sort of thing that happened? [Q]

64. Did you feel there was one doctor who was your particular hospital doctor?
    Yes 4
    No 5
    COMMENTS:
    IF YES (4) Who was that?
    RANK or NAME
    Name known 6
    Name not known 7
    Name forgotten 8

65. Of the doctors you saw while you were actually in hospital—had you seen any of them before in out-patients?
    Yes 9
    No 0
    IF YES (9) Which one(s)?
    RECORD NAME OR RANK

66. Have you seen any of them since you left—in out-patients?
    Yes 1
    No 2
    IF YES (1) Which one(s)?
    RECORD NAME OR RANK

67. In general did the doctors tell you their names when you first saw them—or how did you find them out?
    RECORD COMMENTS AND CODE [Q]
    Doctors introduced themselves . 3
    Patient asked 4
    Nurses told them 5
    Other patients 6
    Other 7

68. Did your own doctor come to visit you at all while you were in hospital?
    Yes 8
    No 9
    IF YES (8)
    (a) Did you talk to him about your illness and treatment?
    Yes 1
    No 2

IF YES (1) Was he able to give you any help-ful explanations?

Yes 3
No 4

IF YES (3) What about? [Q]
(b) What (else) did you discuss? [Q]

IF NO (9)
(a) Would you have liked him to?
RECORD   Yes 5
COMMENTS: No 6
(b) Do you think it would have been helpful if you had been able to discuss your illness and treatment with him while you were in hospital?

Yes 7
No 8

IF YES (7) In what way? [Q]

69. Did you come across any medical students while you were in hospital?

Yes 3
No 4

IF YES (3)
(a) How did you feel about that? [Q]
(b) Can you describe what contact you had with them? [Q]

Now there are one or two questions about your ward and the other patients.

70. How many beds were there in your ward altogether?

1...................... 1
2...................... 2
3...................... 3
4...................... 4
5–9.................... 5
10–14................. 6
15–19................. 7
20–24................. 8
25–9.................. 9
30 +.................. 0

71. Would you have preferred:
OMIT IF ⌠A room of your own 1
SINGLE ⌡A smaller ward 2
ROOM   A larger ward 3
        Ward same size 4
Why is that?

[IF SINGLE ROOM GO ON TO QUESTION 76]

72. Did you feel you had enough privacy?

Yes 5
No 6

IF NO (6) In what way? [Q]

73. Were there curtains round your bed which could be drawn or did they have a movable screen—or what?

Curtains 7
Screen 8
Other (specify) 9

74. Were there any occasions when they did not draw the curtains/move screen round you and you would have liked them to?

Yes 1
No 2

IF YES (1) When was that? [Q]

75. What about the screens/curtains round the other patients—were there any occasions when they were not drawn and you would have liked them to be?

Yes 3
No 4

IF YES (3) When was that? [Q]

[TO ALL]

76 Who did you talk to most while you were in hospital—your visitors, the doctors, the nurses, the other patients—or anyone else?

Visitors 3
Doctors.................... 4
Nurses..................... 5
Patients 6
Other (specify) 7
....

77. What about the other patients. Did you talk to them a great deal, quite a bit or not very much?

A great deal 8
Quite a bit 9
Not very much 0

78. On the whole did you find these discussions:
Very enjoyable.............. 1
PROMPT Fairly enjoyable 2
Not very enjoyable 3

IF NOT VERY ENJOYABLE (3) Why was that? [Q]

79. Did you discuss your illnesses or treatment together a lot, a little or not at all?

A lot 1
A little 2
Not at all 3

IF (1 or 2)
(a) Did you find these discussions at all up-setting? (Sometimes or generally).

Never upsetting 4
Sometimes upsetting......... 5
Generally upsetting.......... 6

IF (5 or 6) In what way? [Q]
(b) Did you find them at all helpful?

Yes 7
No 8

IF YES (7) In what way? [Q]

[IF SINGLE ROOM GO ON TO QUESTION 83]

80. Were there any patients you wished were not in your ward?

Yes 9
No 0

IF YES (9) Why was that?

81. Did any of the illnesses of any of the other patients or the treatment they were having worry or depress you at all?

Yes 1
No 2

IF YES (1) What was the trouble?

82. Do you think some of the patients were too demanding?

Yes 3
No 4

IF YES (3) In what way—can you give me an example?

[TO ALL]

234

83. Did you see the almoner at all while you were in hospital?

Yes 5
No 6

IF YES (5)
(a) What did you see her about? [Q]

(b) Was she able to help you in any way? How? [Q]

IF NO (6) Would you have liked to ask her about anything?

Yes 7
No 8

IF YES (7)
(a) What about?

(b) Why didn't you ask to see her?

84. Occupational status:

Working full time 1
Working part time 2
Retired 3
Housewife not working 4
Temporarily off work because of ill health (specify no. of weeks) . 5
Other (specify) ....

[IF (3 or 4) GO ON TO QUESTION 94]

85. OCCUPATION (TYPE OF WORK) [C]

86. INDUSTRY [C]

87. How long had you been in that job (with that firm)?

Less than 3 months 1
3 months < 6 months 2
6 months < 1 year 3
1 year < 2 years 4
2 years < 5 years 5
5 years < 10 years 6
10 years < 15 years 7
15 years + ... 8

88. Do you think your type of work contributed to your ill health (MATERNITY: affected your health) in any way?

Yes 1
No 2

IF YES (1) How? [Q]

89. Have you now:

Returned to same job 3
Returned to similar job, other employer.................... 4
Returned to other job, same employer.................... 5
Returned to other job, other employer.................... 6
Still off work 7

IF OTHER JOB (5 or 6) Do you think this is more or less suitable for your health?

More 8
Less 9
Same 0

IF OTHER JOB OR EMPLOYER (4, 5 or 6) Do you earn more, less or the same now as you did before?

Now earn more 1
Now earn less 2
Earn same 3
Other (specify) ....

IF RETURNED TO WORK (3, 4, 5 or 6)
(a) How long were you off work altogether?

Less than a week............ 1
1 week < 2 weeks 2
2 weeks < 1 month 3
1 month < 2 months 4
2 months < 3 months 5
3 months < 6 months 6
6 months + (specify no. of months)..................... 7

(b) Do you feel your present job is suitable —as far as your health is concerned?

Yes 1
No 2

IF NO (2) In what way is it not suitable? [Q]

IF STILL OFF WORK
(a) Are you hoping to go back to:

Same job 3
Similar job 4
Other job 5
or what? (specify) ....

(b) Do you think you will have any difficulties? [Q]

90. While you were/are off work did/do you get any wages?

Yes, received full wages 6
Yes, received part wages 7
No 8

IF DID NOT RECEIVE FULL WAGES (7 or 8)
(a) Did you get Sickness Benefit while you were off work?

Yes 9
No 0

IF YES (9) How soon after you went sick did you get your first payment? No. of weeks....
How did you feel about that? [Q]

(b) Did you get any National Assistance?

Yes 1
No 2

(c) Did you get anything from a Union?

Yes 3
No 4

(d) Would you say the loss of your wages was a serious strain on family finances, a moderate strain, a little strain or no strain at all?

Serious strain 5
Moderate strain............. 6
A little strain 7
No strain 8

IF SERIOUS OR MODERATE STRAIN (5 or 6)
How did you manage? [Q and C]

RECAP IF ANY DIFFICULTY ASSOCI-ATED WITH WORK—WORK UNSUIT-ABLE FOR HEALTH, DIFFICULTY FINDING WORK, SERIOUS OR MODER-ATE FINANCIAL STRAIN. IF NOT, GO ON TO Q. 94.

91. Now you've told me about . . . (STATE DIFFICULTY) Did you talk to anyone about this—either at the hospital or since you got home?

Yes 6
No 7

IF YES (6) Who? Anyone else? [C]

Were they able to help you at all?

How? [Q]

92. Did you think about asking any of these people for advice?

	Yes	No	IF YES Why didn't you?
Hospital doctors	1	2	
Sister or nurses	3	4	
Hospital almoner	5	6	
G.P.	7	8	

93. Do you think any of them might have been able to help you?

Yes 9
No 0

IF YES (9)
(a) Who? [C]

(b) Why didn't you ask them? [Q]

94. DETAILS OF PEOPLE LIVING WITH AT TIME OF HOSPITALIZATION

Relationship to Subject	Sex	Age group						Marital status	Occup. status
	M F	Under 2	2 V 5	5 V 10	10 V 15	15 V 65	65 +		Full Part Not
1 SJT.	Y X	see below						S M W D	F P N
2	Y X	1	2	3	4	5	6		F P N
3	Y X	1	2	3	4	5	6		F P N
4	Y X	1	2	3	4	5	6		F P N
5	Y X	1	2	3	4	5	6		F P N
6	Y X	1	2	3	4	5	6		F P N
7	Y X	1	2	3	4	5	6		F P N
8	Y X	1	2	3	4	5	6		F P N
9	Y X	1	2	3	4	5	6		F P N
10	Y X	1	2	3	4	5	6		F P N
11	Y X	1	2	3	4	5	6		F P N

OFF. USE

CHECK: So there are...........altogether

95. How old are you?

21–34	1
35–44	2
45–54	3
55–59	4
60–64	5
65–69	6
70–74	7
75–79	8
80 +	9

96. SUBJECT HOUSEWIFE

Yes 1
No 2

97. SUBJECT HEAD OF HOUSEHOLD

Yes 3
No 4

98. OCCUPATION OF HEAD OF HOUSEHOLD (if not subject) [C]

99. Have you a telephone? (Or is there one you can use if necessary?)

Own phone 3
Access to phone 4
No phone 5

100. ONLY ASK IF SUBJECT LIVES ALONE OR WITH NO ADULT RELATIVES
(a) Who is the relative you see most of? [C]

(b) How often do you see them—on the average?

Every day 5
Once a week or more 6
Once a month 7
Less than once a month....... 8

[(TO ALL]

101. When you left hospital did you go straight to your own home or to a convalescent home or to stay with relatives—or what?

Own home 1
Convalescent home 2
Relatives (specify) 3
....
Other (specify) 4

IF CONVALESCENT HOME (2) What did you think of the convalescent home?

102. Did you feel you were discharged from hospital too soon, about the right time, or do you feel you could have come out earlier—considering both your illness and home circumstances?

Too soon 5
Right time 6
Could have come earlier 7

IF (5 or 7) Why was that?

103. When you first came home did anyone have any time off work or school to look after you?

Yes, time off school 3
Yes, time off work—no money lost 4
Yes, time off work—money lost 5
No 6

104. ONLY ASK IF SUBJECT IS HOUSEWIFE NOT LIVING ALONE
While you were in hospital did anyone have time off work or school to do things in the house?

Yes, time off school 7
Yes, time off work—no money lost 8
Yes, time off work—money lost 9
No 0

Did they have any help from anyone not living here? What about?

	Helped		Nature of help
	Yes	No	
Relatives—own	1	2	
Relatives—in-laws ..	3	4	
Neighbours	5	6	
Home help	7	8	
Anyone else (specify)			

IF MOTHER OF CHILDREN UNDER 15 What happened about the children? [C]

105. IF HOUSEWIFE—WHETHER LIVING ALONE OR NOT
When you got home did you have any more help than usual with the shopping, cooking, cleaning, washing or looking after children?

Yes 1
No 2

IF YES (1)
(a) Who helped?

236

(*b*) What did they help with?

	Shopping	3
CODE	Cooking	4
ALL	Cleaning	5
THAT	Washing	6
APPLY	Looking after children	7

IF NO (2) Could you have done with some?

Yes	8
No	9

IF YES (8) What with?

	Shopping	3
CODE	Cooking	4
ALL	Cleaning	5
THAT	Washing	6
APPLY	Looking after children	7

[TO ALL]

106. Have you had any help from a district nurse, home help, health visitor, or anyone like that since you left hospital?

No	1
Yes, district nurse	2
Yes, home help	3
Yes, health visitor	4
Other (specify)	5

....
IF YES (2, 3, 4 or 5)
(*a*) How did that work?

(*b*) Who arranged that?

IF NO (1) Do you think any of those people could have helped you?

Yes	5
No	6

IF YES (5)
(*a*) Who?

(*b*) How?

107. How long have you been out of hospital now?

Less than 2 weeks	1
2 weeks < 1 month	2
1 month < 2 months	3
2 months < 3 months	4
3 months < 4 months	5
4 months < 5 months	6
5 months or more	7

108. How soon after you came out of hospital did you see your own doctor, G.P.?

Within 3 days	8
3 days < 1 week	9
1 week < 2 weeks	0
2 weeks < 1 month	1
1 month < 3 months	2
3 months + (specify)	3
Not seen	4

IF SEEN
(*a*) Is that the same doctor as you had before you went into hospital?

Yes	5
No	6

IF NO (6) Why did you change?

(*b*) Are you satisfied that the doctor was told all he needed to know about your condition by the hospital?

Yes	7
No	8

COMMENTS: [Q]

109. Who do you find it easier to talk to—your own doctor or the doctors in the hospital?

G.P. easier to talk to	7
Hospital doctors easier to talk to	8
No difference	9
Other......................	0

IF PREFERENCE EXPRESSED (7 or 8)
Why is that, do you think? [Q]

110. Who do you feel knows most about your *general* health—your own doctor or one of the hospital doctors?

G.P. knows most	1
Hospital doctor knows most ..	2
No difference	3
Other......................	4

COMMENTS:
IF HOSPITAL DOCTOR (2) Which one?
RECORD NAME (OR RANK)

111. When you left hospital did they give you any advice or instructions or tell you not to do certain things?

Yes	5
No	5

IF YES (5)
(*a*) What? Anything else? RECORD DETAILS AND CODE

	Medicines	1
	Exercises	2
CODE	Diet	3
ALL	Cut down/stop smoking	4
THAT	Take it easy/don't overdo it	5
APPLY	Rest	6
	Take holiday	7
	Not lift heavy things	8
	Other......................	9

(*b*) Who suggested that?
RECORD RANK OR NAME IF DOCTOR
....

Sister	0
Nurse	1
Almoner	2
Physiotherapist	3
Other (specify)	

(*c*) Have you been able to carry it out?

Yes	1
No	2

IF NO (2) What was the difficulty?

(*d*) Do you think it was helpful advice?

Yes	3
No	4

IF NO (4) Why not?

112. Would you have liked any advice (about anything else)?

Yes	5
No	6

IF YES (5) What about?

113. When you left hospital did you have to go back there as an out-patient?

Yes	5
No	6

IF YES (5)
(*a*) Are you still attending out-patients?

Yes	7
No	8

(*b*) How many times have you been back altogether?
NUMBER ....
IF MORE THAN ONCE. As far as you can tell is/was it really necessary for you to go back to hospital or could your own doctor have done everything that was necessary for you? RECORD COMMENTS AND CODE [Q]

Hospital necessary	9
G.P. could do it	0

IF G.P. COULD DO IT. Which would you prefer—to go to the hospital or to your own doctor.

Prefer hospital	1
Prefer G.P.	2
Qualified	3

Why is that?

237

114. If you had the sort of illness which, from a medical point of view, could be treated either at home or in hospital, which would you prefer?
    Prefer home 4
    Prefer hospital 5
    Why is that? [Q & C]

[PRIVATE HOSPITAL PATIENTS ASK QUESTIONS 115–121. OTHERS GO ON TO QUESTION 122]

115. Why did you go as a private patient instead of going under the N.H.S.? [Q]

116. Do you have an insurance scheme for private medical care?
    Yes 2
    No 3
    IF YES (2) Why is that?

117. Did you consider the possibility of an amenity bed?

118. Did you know of the existence of amenity beds?
    Yes 4
    No 5

119. Do you know if there were any amenity beds available?
    Yes, available 6
    No, not available 7
    Don't know 8

120. How much did it cost?

	Total cost	Amount covered by Insurance	Amount paid by patient
(a) For the hospital			
(b) For medical fees and treatment			

121. Do you think it was worth it?
    Yes 9
    No 0
    IF YES (9) In what way? [Q]

    IF NO (0) Why not? [Q]

[TO ALL]
122. Three final questions—what would you say was your worst experience while you were in hospital?

123. Would you say your hospital treatment was:
    Completely successful 1
    PROMPT Partially successful 2
    or Unsuccessful 3
    IF (2 or 3) In what way?

124. I've asked a lot of questions about different things related to your experience in hospital—is there anything else that you feel is interesting or important from the patient's point of view that you would like to tell me.
    THANK INFORMANT. LEAVE LEAFLET

125. Date of interview   /   /

126. Interviewer

127. INTERVIEWER'S ASSESSMENT
    Informant particularly helpful . 1
    Informant reasonably helpful .. 2
    Informant not very helpful 3
    IF (1 or 3) Give possible reason:

128. INTERVIEWER'S ASSESSMENT
    Particularly revealing interview 4
    Average interview 5
    Rather superficial interview 6
    IF (4 or 6) Give reason:

129. Any points of particular interest arising in interview.

Interview Schedules

INTRODUCTION: I explained in my letter that this study is financed by the Nuffield Provincial Hospitals Trust and that we are interested in the relationship between hospitals and general practitioners and between hospitals and patients. We want to obtain the views of a representative sample of general practitioners on this subject. All replies are treated as confidential and of course no names are ever quoted in our reports. When we include a quotation from an interview we make quite sure it's not possible to identify the person who made it. Is there anything more you want to know about the study at this stage—or shall I go ahead and ask you my questions, then you will see what it is all about and you can ask me about any particular points as we go along.

1. Do you hold a hospital appointment?

Yes 1
No 2

IF YES (1)
(a) Hospital

(b) Appointment

(c) Speciality

(d) What proportion of your time does it take up—compared with your general practice?

10% or less	3
Over 10%—25%	4
HOSPITAL Over 25%—33%	5
Over 33%—50%	6
Over 50%—67%	7
Over 67%—75%	8
Over 75%	9

(e) How do you find this works?
Advantages
Any disadvantages
IF NO (2) Would you like to do so?

Yes 3
No 4

IF YES (3) What appointment would you like to hold?
RANK:
SPECIALITY:
IF NO (4) Why not?

2. What do you feel about the relationship between general practitioners and hospitals in this particular area.

3. Have you any suggestions about anything that could be done to improve the relationship in this particular area?

Yes 5
No 6

IF YES (5) What? Anything else?

4. What do you think about the length of time your patients have to wait before they are seen by the hospital—or before they are admitted?

5. Are there any groups of patients—or types of cases—that you have particular difficulty in getting seen or admitted?

Yes 5
No 6

IF YES (5) Which?

6. Do you think the hospitals themselves are sufficiently aware of this problem?

Yes 7
COMMENTS: No 8
Qual. 9

7. Do you have direct access to any of these facilities:

	Yes	No
Routine chest X-rays	1	3
Other X-rays	2	5
Barium meals......	0	0
Pathological tests ..	4	6
Bacteriological tests	7	8

Are you satisfied with the provision of these services in this area?

Yes 1
No 2

IF NO (2) In what way?

Is there anything else you would like direct access to?

8. What do you feel about the ways in which hospitals keep G.P.s informed about their patients' progress and the treatment and investigation which is being carried out?

9. In general would you say you are given enough information about this?

Yes 7
No 8

IF YES (7) Always or usually?

Always 9
Usually 0

IF NO (8) or USUALLY (0)
(a) What type of information do you feel you need more of?

(b) Can you give me an illustration of a case when you would have liked more information?

10. Do you think the hospitals sometimes send you too much detail?

Yes 1
No 2

IF YES (1) Can you give me an example of that?

11. Do you feel you generally receive the information soon enough?

Yes 3
No 4

IF YES (3) Always or usually?

Always 5
Usually 6

IF NO (4) or USUALLY (6) In what sort of situation do you feel this?

12. Do you generally know when a patient has been or is about to be admitted—in time to visit him in hospital if you wanted to? Always or generally?

No 7
Always 8
Generally 9

IF ALWAYS OR GENERALLY (8 or 9)
Who do you hear this from most often?

Hospital 1
Patients 2
Relatives 3

COMMENTS:

13. What do you feel about domiciliary consultations?

14. (a) In what way do you find them most useful?

(b) Do you ever use them for getting patients admitted?

15. How many have you had in the last twelve months?

16. Have you always been able to go there with the consultant?

Yes 5
No 6
COMMENTS:

17. It has been suggested that it would be helpful if consultants could ask G.P.s to go to hospital sometimes for a hospital consultation when the patient is in hospital. What do you feel about that?

18. Can you give me an example of any occasion on which you feel it would have been helpful if a consultant had asked you to come and discuss one of your patients with him, while they were in hospital:

19. Do you think hospital doctors are sufficiently aware of the problems of general practice or do you think it would be helpful if they had more experience of general practice work?

Sufficiently aware 7
More experience would help ... 8
Other (specify) ....
IF MORE EXPERIENCE WOULD HELP
(8) In what way do you think it would affect the relationship between G.P.s and hospitals?

20. How well would you say you know most of the consultants to whom you refer your patients?

IF ANY KNOWN
(a) How did you get to know them initially?

21. Do you think you have enough (Would you like some?) personal contact with them—or with other hospital staff?

22. What do you feel about G.P.s visiting their patients when they are in hospital?

23. Have you visited any of yours in the last four weeks?

Number ....
How many would you say you had visited in the last twelve months?

Number ....

24. Would you like to do this more often?

25. When you go, do you feel the hospital staff welcome your visit, resent it or are indifferent? If you went what do you think the hospital staff would welcome your visit, resent it or be indifferent?

Welcome.................... 5
Resent 6
Indifferent 7
COMMENTS:

26. IF VISITED SIX OR MORE IN YEAR
(a) Who do you normally see on the hospital staff when you visit your patients?

(b) Are there any particular groups of patients or type of cases that you make a particular point of visiting?

27. I'd like to ask you about the amount of information you think doctors should give their patients—about their illness and treatment. Apart from the problem of people with fatal illnesses, how much do you think patients should be told?

28. Here are two statements—would you read them and tell me which one most nearly describes your own views.
STATEMENT 1
Since patients often have difficulty in formulating the questions they want to ask, doctors should anticipate their needs and explain their illness, their treatment and their progress to them as fully as possible in terms they can understand.
STATEMENT 2
Doctors should explain to their patients as much as it is necessary for them to know about their illness, treatment and progress in order that they can co-operate as fully as possible with the doctor in the treatment.

Statement 1
Statement 2

29. Is there any modification or qualification you would like to make to that statement?

30. Do you think hospitals keep patients reasonably informed in this way about their illnesses and the treatment they receive?

31. If there was a closer or more intimate contact between G.P.s and hospitals do you think G.P.s could help to keep hospital patients better informed about things—or do you think there is little room for improvement or do you think hospitals should improve their way of handling this on their own?

G.P.s could help 3
No need for improvement 4
Hospitals should improve on own 2
COMMENTS:

32. Would you say you are satisfied or dissatisfied with the N.H.S. conditions under which you treat your patients?

Satisfied 6
Dissatisfied 7
IF SATISFIED (6)
Any suggestions for improvements?

IF DISSATISFIED (7)
(a) In what way?

(b) What do you think could be done in order to help you with this?

Any other comments on the hospital service and relationship between G.P.s and hospitals?

33. Are you in partnership?
    Yes 1
    No 2
    IF YES (1) How many partners are there—including you?

    ....

34. Do you have an assistant?
    Yes 3
    No 4

35. Do you have a trainee?
    Yes 5
    No 6

36. Do you have a secretary or nurse?
    Secretary.................... 1
    Nurse 2
    Neither 3

37. How many patients do you have on your list?
    IF IN PARTNERSHIP—that is the number on which your superannuation is calculated:
    Up to 1,500 5
    1,501–2,000 6
    2,001–2,500 7
    2,501–3,000 8
    3,001 or more 9

Date of interview .... / /

Time of interview ....

Interviewer ....

We would like to have a picture of the nature and frequency of all the different sorts of contacts that general practitioners have with hospitals. Would you be willing, for one week, to keep a record for us of all your contacts—that is letters, phone calls and visits? I have a recording sheet made up which shows just what we want you to put down.

Agreed to keep diary Yes 4
No 5

How long have you been working in this practice?

241

APPENDIX 4

THE TWELVE STUDY AREAS

THE twelve constituencies in which this inquiry was made have been described in the introduction. They were considered in five groups:
(1) Middle-class town-and-country districts (with expanding populations).

TABLE M. CHARACTERISTICS OF

Constituency		Population 1961	Population changes		Area sq. miles	Proportion in rural districts
			1951–61	1931–51		
Middle-class town and country districts with expanding populations	Lewes	80,123	17·4%	24·2%	152	43%
	Melton	109,875	24·9%	26·1%	349	85%
	St. Albans	82,262	21·6%	54·7%	49	32%
Middle-class urban areas with static populations	Wallasey	103,213	1·8%	3·1%	9	None
	Wimbledon	56,994	−2·0%	−2·3%	5	None
Agricultural area	Torrington	62,110	−1·3%	3·7%	583	55%
Working-class towns	Durham	92,080	0·9%	−1·8%	79	37%
	Leigh	82,721	−5·4%	3·2%	22	None
	Pontypool	69,993	6·6%	−1·6%	41	None
Working-class city districts	Birmingham Sparkbrook		(−0·6%)	(11·0%)		None
	Lambeth Vauxhall		(−3·1%)	(−22·3%)		None
	Sunderland North		(4·5%)	(−2·4%)		None

Figures in brackets relate to the administrative area of which the constituency is a part. Lambeth Vauxhall is one of the three, Sunderland North one of two

(2) Middle-class urban areas (with static populations).

(3) Agricultural.

(4) Working-class towns.

(5) Working-class city districts.

The various factors which were taken into account in grouping the constituencies are shown in Table M.

THE TWELVE STUDY AREAS

Proportion aged 65+ (1951)	Politics			Proportion of jurors on electoral register (1954)	Social Class (1951)	
	M.P. 1959	*Majority*	*M.P.* 1945–59		*I and II*	*IV and V*
15·3%	Conservative	16,577	Conservative	10·0%	26·1%	28·4%
10·7%	Conservative	12,821	Conservative	9·4%	20·6%	28·6%
9·9%	Conservative	8,507	Lab./Con.	10·5%	22·5%	23·5%
12·1%	Conservative	15,066	Conservative	10·5%	23·0%	23·2%
14·4%	Conservative	10,860	Conservative	10·6%	30·7%	17·4%
14·3%	Conservative	2,265 over Lib.	Lib./Con.	3·8%	30·0%	32·5%
9·4%	Labour	16,689	Labour	1·9%	10·9%	40·2%
9·6%	Labour	14,775	Labour	1·2%	10·0%	38·8%
9·9%	Labour	17,852	Labour	0·3%	9·8%	40·8%
(9·3%)	Conservative	886	Labour	2·1%	(13·7%)	(27·3%)
(11·0%)	Labour	7,125	Labour	3·0%	(13·6%)	(28·7%)
(9·2%)	Labour	2,208	Labour	1·5%	(11·5%)	(34·0%)

and Birmingham Sparkbrook one of 13 constituencies in the larger administrative districts for which Census Data are available.

243

Appendix 4

Some comparisons between middle- and working-class areas have been made in the chapter describing social class variations. Some of the other differences between the areas are discussed in this appendix.

Hospitalization rates

Estimated hospitalization rates in the six-month study period varied in the twelve areas from 28 to 52 per 1,000 population (Table N).

Hospitalization rates were highest in Lambeth Vauxhall and Wimbledon—two of the three areas in which 30% or more of the patients had been in teaching hospitals. Analysis by the proportion of people aged 65 or more, and by social class indices, revealed no significant correlations with hospitalization rates. But areas in which the population had expanded greatly between 1931 and 1961 have a lower hospitalization rate than those in which the population had contracted or remained the same. The rate of expansion of the populations in the twelve areas over the period 1931–61 is negatively related to hospitalization rates (r = −0·65, ·02 <p< ·05). This association is shown in Fig. 1.

Between 1931 and 1961 the amount of hospital building was negligible, and it might perhaps be expected that in areas where the population had

TABLE N

HOSPITALIZATION RATES IN TWELVE STUDY AREAS

		Estimated six-monthly hospitalization rate per 1,000 population
Middle-class town-and-country districts (with expanding populations)	Lewes Melton St. Albans	42 34 } 35 28
Middle-class urban areas (with static populations)	Wallasey Wimbledon	43 51 } 46
Agricultural area	Torrington	41 41
Working-class towns	Durham Leigh Pontypool	42 35 } 37 30

Working-class city districts	Birmingham
	  Sparkbrook
	Lambeth
	  Vauxhall
	Sunderland
	  North
		36
		
		52 } 45
		
		47

The Twelve Study Areas

expanded rapidly the number of hospital beds available would be lower, per head of population, than in areas where the population had remained static or even declined. One of the difficulties in testing such a hypothesis is to decide what type and size of area it is most appropriate to study. Hospital catchment areas are not defined, geographically or administratively, and if sizeable towns are considered their hospitals may serve a large surrounding area where patterns of population movement have been different from those in the town itself. An analysis of the 38 County Boroughs for which hospitalization rates are given in the Ministry of Health and General Register Office 1958 study[1] did not show any consistent relationship with population changes. It is, however, possible that constituencies are slightly more appropriate areas to study in this context, so it will be interesting to see what emerges from the further analyses of the official inquiry.

FIGURE 1

THE ASSOCIATION BETWEEN POPULATION CHANGES AND
HOSPITALIZATION RATE

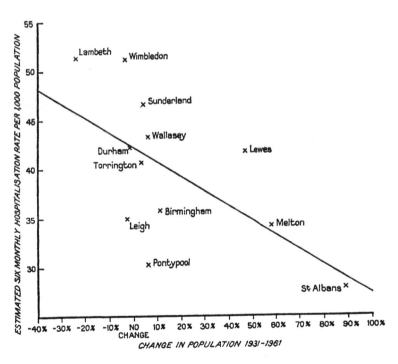

[1] Ministry of Health and General Register Office, *Report on Hospital In-patient Enquiry for the Year 1958: Part II.*

245

Appendix 4

It might be argued that the comparatively low hospitalization rate found, in the present study, in expanding areas reflects differences in morbidity—mobile people being less likely to need hospital care than others. But Table O shows that waiting times are greater in areas where the

TABLE O

DELAYS FOR WAITING-LIST ADMISSIONS AND HOSPITALIZATION RATE IN AREA

Estimated six-monthly hospitalization rate per 1,000 population	Areas included. (hospitalization rate in brackets)	Proportion waiting a month or more before being seen at out-patients	Proportion waiting three months or more before admission	Number of patients ($= 100\%$)
45 or more	Lambeth V. (52) Wimbledon (51) Sunderland N. (47)	6%	14%	85
40 or more but less than 45	Wallasey (43) Durham (42) Lewes (42) Torrington (41)	13%	19%	125
Under 40	B'ham S. (36) Leigh (35) Melton (34) Pontypool (30) St. Albans (28)	20%	21%	133

hospitalization rate is low; this suggests that pressure on beds is greater and that part of the difference at any rate is due simply to lack of hospital space.

The proportion of waiting-list admissions in our survey who had to wait for a month or more before being seen at an out-patient department was 6% in areas where the hospitalization rate was high (over 45 per 1,000), and 20% in those where it was low (40 or less). Variations in the delay between being seen at the out-patient department and admitted to hospital are in the same direction, but are not so marked. There did not, however, appear to be any direct relationship in the study areas between hospitalization rates and length of stay, the proportion of maternity cases or the proportion of general practitioner referrals which were admitted directly.

Summary and conclusions

To sort out the complex relationships between the various social characteristics of the areas and the different indices of hospital care, it would be necessary to study many more areas and to apply much more elaborate and sophisticated statistical techniques. Simple analysis of the limited data from this inquiry suggests that hospitalization rates are comparatively high in areas served by teaching hospitals and relatively low in districts where the population has expanded a great deal in the last 30 years. There is some evidence that a low hospitalization rate is associated with comparatively long delays, but this association is not so strong as might perhaps be expected. This indicates that some of the variations in the availability of hospital beds may be a reflection of the needs of the area, or that the community has adjusted its demands to the facilities available.

APPENDIX 5

STATISTICAL SIGNIFICANCE

THERE has been some discussion about the applicability of statistical tests of significance to social studies of this kind. A number of American sociologists[1] have attacked their use.

I recognize that there are many factors, particularly the nature of the data and the stage at which hypotheses are often formulated, which violate some of the conditions in which these tests apply and make their interpretation difficult. For this reason no mention of them has been made in the text, in an attempt to avoid the appearance of spurious precision which the presentation of such tests might seem to imply. Nevertheless, until more appropriate techniques are developed, I feel these tests provide some indication of the probability of differences occurring by chance. In fact, χ^2 tests have been applied constantly when looking at the data from this survey and have influenced decisions about what differences to present and how much verbal 'weight' to attach to them. In general, attention has not been drawn to any difference which statistical tests suggest might have occurred by chance five or more times in 100.

[1] Selvin, H. C., 'A Critique of Tests of Significance in Survey Research' Lipset, S. M., Trow, M. A., and Coleman, J. S., *Union Democracy*, Appendix I, Methodological Note.

APPENDIX 6

CLASSIFICATION OF SOCIAL CLASS

THE classification used is based on the Registrar-General's Classification of Occupations (1960).[1] This distinguishes five 'social classes':

I Professional, etc., occupations.
II Intermediate occupations.
III Skilled occupations.
IV Partly skilled occupations.
V Unskilled occupations.

These classes are intended to reflect 'the general standing within the community of the occupations concerned'. Occupations in classes II, III and IV are also classified as 'manual', 'non-manual' or 'agricultural'. In the analyses here these five classes are used, but Class III, skilled occupations, is divided into manual and non-manual groups to give a six-point scale. In a number of instances the main differences that emerge are between what can be described as the 'middle class' and 'working class', the former being most of the non-manual occupations—the Registrar-General's social classes I, II and III non-manual—and the latter almost entirely manual—

TABLE P

PATIENTS' SOCIAL CLASS

	%	
Middle class		
Professional	4	⎫
Intermediate	18	⎬ 33
Skilled non-manual	11	⎭
Working class		
Skilled manual	38	⎫
Partly skilled	21	⎬ 67
Unskilled	8	⎭
Number of patients* (= 100%)	685	

* The 54 patients for whom inadequate information was obtained have been excluded.

[1] General Register Office, *Classification of Occupations 1960*.

249

III manual, IV and V. Table P shows the proportion of patients in these groups. Men and single women have been classified on the basis of their present occupation if they were under 60, or on their main occupation if they were aged 60 or more. Married and widowed women have been classified according to their husband's present, last or main occupation.

APPENDIX 7

REFERENCES

BACKETT, E. M. 'Future Role of the Family Doctor'. *Lancet*, ii, p. 1075. 1960.

BANTON, M. *White and Coloured*. London, Jonathan Cape. 1959.

BARR, A. 'Training of Student Nurses'. *Brit. J. prev. soc. Med.* Vol. XIII, p. 149. 1959.

BARTON, R. *Institutional Neurosis*. Bristol, John Wright. 1959.

BRAINE, B. in *Hansard*. Vol. 673, No. 74, col 957. 1963.

BROTHERSTON, J. H. F. 'Towards New Incentives'. *Lancet*, i, p. 1119. 1963.

CARMICHAEL, L., ROSS, F., and STEVENSON, J. S. K. 'Why Are They Waiting?: a Survey of Out-patient Referrals'. *Brit. med. J.*, i, p. 736. 1963.

CAUTER, T., and DOWNHAM, J. S. *The Communication of Ideas*. London, Chatto and Windus. 1954.

COLE, D., with UTTING, J. *The Economic Circumstances of Old People*. Occasional Papers on Social Administration. No. 4. Welwyn, Codicote Press. 1962.

COSER, R. L. 'A Home Away from Home.' *Sociological Studies of Health and Sickness* edited by Dorian Apple. New York, McGraw-Hill Book Co., p. 168. 1962.

COUNCIL OF THE COLLEGE OF GENERAL PRACTITIONERS. 'Content of General Practice'. *Lancet*, ii, p. 1108. 1962.

COUNCIL OF THE INSTITUTE OF ALMONERS. *Medical Social Work: a Statement on the Organization and Function of an Almoner's Department.* London, Institute of Almoners. 1958.

CROSS, K. W., and HALL, D. L. A. 'Survey of Entrants to Nurse Training Schools and of Student-nurse Wastage in the Birmingham Region'. *Brit. J. prev. soc. Med.* Vol. VIII, p. 70. 1954.

CURRAN, A. P., and FERGUSON, T. *Further Studies in Hospital and Community*. London, Oxford University Press. 1962.

DEWAR, R., and SOMMER, R. 'Disturbing Noise in a Mental Hospital'. *Brit. Med. J.*, i. p. 1566. 1960.

FERGUSON, T., and MACPHAIL, A. N. *Hospital and Community*. London, Oxford University Press. 1954.

FORSYTH, G., and LOGAN, R. F. L. *The Demand for Medical Care*. London, Oxford University Press. 1960.

FOX, T. F. 'The Personal Doctor and His Relation to the Hospital'. *Lancet*, i, p. 743. 1960.

FREIDSON, E. *Patients' Views of Medical Practice*. New York, Russell Sage Foundation. 1961.

GEFFEN, D. H., and WARREN, M. D. 'The Care of the Aged'. *Med. Offr.* Vol. 91, p. 285. 1954.

Appendix 7

GENERAL REGISTER OFFICE. *Classification of Occupations 1960*. London, H.M.S.O. 1960.

GENERAL REGISTER OFFICE. *Statistical Review of England and Wales for the Year 1959. Supplement on Mental Health*. London, H.M.S.O. 1962.

GRAY, P. G., CORLETT, T., and JONES, P. *The Proportion of Jurors as an Index of the Economic Status of a District*. London, The Social Survey. 1951.

HALL., J., and JONES, D. C. 'Social Grading of Occupations'. *Brit. J. Sociol.* Vol. I, No. 1, p. 51. 1950.

HAYWOOD, S. C., JEFFORD, R. E., MacGREGOR, R. B. K., STEVENSON, K., and WOODING JONES, G. D. E. 'The Patient's View of the Hospital'. *The Hospital*. Vol. 57, p. 644. 1961.

HORDER, E. 'The Care of the Elderly'. *Practitioner*. Vol. 189, p. 648. 1962.

Hospital and Social Services Journal. 'Nurse Training—Proposed Common Portal Experiment in Sheffield Region'. p. 1315. November 1962.

HUGHES, H. L. G. *Peace at the Last*. London, Calouste Gulbenkian Foundation. 1960.

IRVINE, R. E., and SMITH, B. J. 'Patterns of Visiting', *Lancet*, i, p. 597. 1963.

JARRETT, R. J., and GAZET, J- C. 'Aspects of Convalescence after Herniorrhaphy'. *Brit. med. J.*, i, p. 930. 1961.

JOINT SUB-COMMITTEE OF THE STANDING MEDICAL AND STANDING NURSING ADVISORY COMMITTEES FOR THE CENTRAL HEALTH SERVICES COUNCIL AND THE MINISTER OF HEALTH. *Communication between Doctors, Nurses and Patients*. London, H.M.S.O. 1963.

Lancet. 'Annotation'. i, p. 957. 1962.

LEE, J. A. H., MORRISON, S. L., and MORRIS, J. N. 'Fatality from Three Common Surgical Conditions in Teaching and Non-Teaching Hospitals'. *Lancet*, ii, p. 785. 1957.

LEE, J. A. H., MORRISON, S. L., and MORRIS, J. N. 'Case-Fatality in Teaching and Non-Teaching Hospitals'. *Lancet*, i, p. 170. 1960.

LIPSET, S. M., TROW, M. A., and COLEMAN, J. S. *Union Democracy*. Glencoe, Ill., Free Press. 1956.

McGHEE, A. *The Patient's Attitude to Nursing Care*. Edinburgh and London, E. & S. Livingstone. 1961.

McKEOWN, T. 'The Future of Medical Practice outside the Hospital'. *Lancet*, i, p. 923. 1962.

MEDICAL DEFENCE UNION AND ROYAL COLLEGE OF NURSING. *Joint Memorandum on Steps that Might be taken to Obviate the Risk of an Operation being Performed on the Wrong Patient, Side, Limb or Digit*. London, Royal College of Nursing. 1961.

MEDICAL SERVICES REVIEW COMMITTEE. *A Review of the Medical Services in Great Britain*. London, Social Assay. 1962.

MILNE, J. F. (Ed.) *The Hospitals Year Book 1961*. London, Institute of Hospital Administrators. 1960.

MINISTRY OF HEALTH. *A Hospital Plan for England and Wales*. Cmnd. 1604. London, H.M.S.O. 1962.

MINISTRY OF HEALTH. *Circular on Visiting of Patients*. H.M. (62) 39. London, H.M.S.O. 1962.

252

References

MINISTRY OF HEALTH. *Report for the Year 1952, Part II.* Cmnd. 9009. London, H.M.S.O. 1953.

MINISTRY OF HEALTH. *Report for the Year 1961, Part I.* Cmnd. 1754. London, H.M.S.O. 1962.

MINISTRY OF HEALTH AND GENERAL REGISTER OFFICE. *Report on Hospital In-patient Enquiry for the Year 1958, Part II.* London, H.M.S.O. 1961.

MINISTRY OF HEALTH AND GENERAL REGISTER OFFICE. *Report on Hospital In-patient Enquiry for the Year 1960, Part II.* London, H.M.S.O. 1963.

NATIONAL BIRTHDAY TRUST FUND. 'Perinatal Mortality Survey'. Summary in *Brit. med. J.*, ii, p. 1187. 1962.

NUFFIELD PROVINCIAL HOSPITALS TRUST. *The Work of Nurses in Hospital Wards.* London, Oxford University Press. 1953.

NUFFIELD PROVINCIAL HOSPITALS TRUST. *Studies in the Functions and Design of Hospitals.* London, Oxford University Press. 1955.

Nursing Times. 'Student Nurse Wastage, East Anglia'. Vol. 50, p. 921. 1954.

OXFORD AREA NURSE TRAINING COMMITTEE. *From Student to Nurse.* Oxford, Area Nurse Training Committee. 1961.

PEP. *Family Needs and the Social Services.* London, Allen and Unwin. 1961.

PLATT, B. S., EDDY, T. P., and PELLETT, P. L. *Food in Hospitals.* London, Oxford University Press. 1963.

PRATT, L., SELIGMANN, A., and READER, G. 'Physicians' Views on the Level of Medical Information among Patients'. *Amer. J. publ. Hlth.* Vol. 47, p. 1277. 1957.

REVANS, R. W. 'Hospital Attitudes and Communications'. *Sociol. Rev.* Monograph No. 5, p. 117. 1962.

REVANS, R. W. 'The Hospital as a Human System'. *Physics in Medicine and Biology.* Vol. 7, p. 147. 1962.

SCOTT, C. 'Research on Mail Surveys'. *J. R. statist. Soc.* Series A. Vol. 124, p. 143. 1961.

SELVIN, H. C. 'A Critique of Tests of Significance in Survey Research'. *Amer. sociol. Rev.* Vol. 22, p. 519. 1957.

SPROTT, W. J. H. *Human Groups.* London, Penguin Books. 1958.

SUSSER, M. W., and WATSON, W. *Sociology in Medicine.* London, Oxford University Press. 1962.

STATHAM, C. 'Noise and the Patient in Hospital'. *Brit. med. J.*, ii, p. 1247. 1959.

TITMUSS, R. M. *Essays on the Welfare State.* London, Allen and Unwin. 1958.

TOWNSEND, P. *The Family Life of Old People.* London, Routledge and Kegan Paul. 1957. Pelican Books. 1963.

WALLACE, C. P. Presidential address to the Surrey Branch of the B.M.A. Reported in *Brit. med. J. suppl.*, ii, p. 3014. 1962.

WILLCOCK, H. D. *Nursing Methods in a General Hospital.* London, Central Office of Information. SS.251. 1961.

WILLMOTT, P., and P. 'Off Work through Illness'. *New Society.* Vol. I, No. 15. 1963.

WILLMOTT, P., and YOUNG, M. *Family and Class in a London Suburb.* London, Routledge and Kegan Paul. 1960.

WORKING PARTY ON THE RECRUITMENT AND TRAINING OF NURSES. *Report.* London, H.M.S.O. 1947.

WORLD HEALTH ORGANIZATION. *Manual of the International Statistical Classification of Diseases, Injuries, and Causes of Death.* London, H.M.S.O. 1957.

WRIGHT, M. S. *A Study of the Characteristics of Successful and Unsuccessful Student Nurses in Scotland.* Edinburgh, University. 1961.

YOUNG, M., and WILLMOTT, P. 'Social Grading by Manual Workers'. *Brit. J. Sociol.* Vol. VII. No. 4, p. 337. 1956.

YOUNG, M., and WILLMOTT, P. *Family and Kinship in East London.* London, Routledge and Kegan Paul. 1957. Pelican Books. 1962.

INDEX

Abel-Smith, B., 203n
Administrators, 203
Admission to hospital, 12–30 *passim* 189, 192, 200, 203, 246
Age of patients; 8, 219, and contact with almoner, 163
and information, 80–1, 177
and presence of husband during labour, 141–2
and privacy, 186–7
people who live alone, 148–50
proportion blaming job for ill-health, 159
proportion in teaching hospitals, 170
relationship with nurses, 179
relationship with other patients, 184–7
telephone, 149
visiting, 149
See also Old people
Agricultural area, 7, 242–3
Almoners; 98, 162–4, 174
Council of the Institute of, 162n
Anaesthetist, patients' contact with, 95–6, 173, 175, 189
Areas, *see* Study areas
Atherton, 7

Babies, *see* Maternity patients
Backett, E. M., 15
Banton, M., 194
Barr, A., 44
Barrow-upon-Soar, 6
Barton, R., 185
Bed-making, and hospital routine, 40, 46
Bed-pans and bottles; and other patients, 55
difficulty in obtaining, 36

lack of privacy when using, 56, 58
Belvoir, 6
Bideford, 7
Billesdon, 6
Birmingham Sparkbrook, 7–8, 173, 190, 200, 209, 210, 213, 214, 242–6
Blaenavon, 7
Braine, B., 97n
Breast-feeding, 184
Brighton, 6
Brotherston, J. H. F., 205n
Burgess Hill, 6

Carmichael, L., 25n
Casualty departments, 21
Cauter, T., 184
Children; and contact with people who live alone, 149
and visiting, 137
care of, when mother in hospital, 142–3
care of, when mother comes out of hospital, 145–6
time off school, while mother in hospital, 143, 198
Class, *see* Social class
Clinical assistants, 87, 92, 109, 178
Clinics, maternity and child welfare, 21
Cole, D., 154n
Coleman, J. S., 248n
College of General Practitioners, 119
Coloured nurses *see* Nurses, coloured
Communication, problem of, 73–115 *passim*, 175
See also Information

255

Index

257

Index

Welfare services, and the almoner, 162–4
Wheathampstead, 6
Willcock, H. D., 33n, 38n
Willmott, P., and P., 154n
Willmott, P., 82n, 142n, 184, 198n
Wimbledon, 6, 173, 190, 200, 209, 213, 214, 242, 244–6
Wirral, 6
Wooding Jones, G. D. E., 61n
Work, 8, 14, 25, 152–62 *passim*

Working-class; city-districts, 7–8, 242–4
towns, 7, 242–4
See also Social class for comparisons with middle-class
Working Party on the Recruitment and Training of Nurses, 44
World Health Organization, 9
Wright, M. S., 44

Young M., 82n, 142n, 184, 198n

For Product Safety Concerns and Information please contact our EU
representative GPSR@taylorandfrancis.com
Taylor & Francis Verlag GmbH, Kaufingerstraße 24, 80331 München, Germany

www.ingramcontent.com/pod-product-compliance
Ingram Content Group UK Ltd.
Pitfield, Milton Keynes, MK11 3LW, UK
UKHW021111180425
457613UK00005B/47